THE PICTURE OF HEALTH®

DAILY POWER PLAN™
100-DAY DEVOTIONAL

DAILY WALKS WITH GOD TO EXERCISE YOUR FAITH AND HEAL YOUR BODY

DR. RAY AND MICHELLE PEARSON

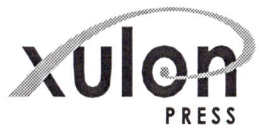

Copyright © 2007 by Dr. Ray and Michelle Pearson

The Picture of Health Daily Power Plan 100-day Devotional
by Dr. Ray and Michelle Pearson

Printed in the United States of America

ISBN 978-1-60266-035-9

All rights reserved solely by the author. The author guarantees all contents are original and do not infringe upon the legal rights of any other person or work. No part of this book may be reproduced in any form without the permission of the author. The views expressed in this book are not necessarily those of the publisher.

Unless otherwise indicated all scriptures are from the New International Version (NIV) Copyright © 1973, 1978, 1984 by International Bible Society, used by permission.

Other versions cited are: King James Version of the Bible (KJV), Public Domain; Amplified Bible (AMP) Copyright © 1954, 1958, 1962, 1964, 1965, 1987 by The Lockman Foundation, used by permission; New Living Translation (NLT) © 1996 by Tyndale Charitable Trust. Used by permission of Tyndale House Publishers; (The Message) © 1993, 1994, 1995, 1996, 2000, 2001, 2002 by Eugene H. Peterson; (NKJV) New King James Version Copyright © 1982 by Thomas Nelson, Inc.; The Bible text designated (YLT) is from the 1898 Young's Literal Translation by Robert Young, Public Domain; English Standard Version (ESV) The Holy Bible, English Standard Version Copyright © 2001 by Crossway Bibles, a division of Good News Publishers; RVR1960 Copyright © 1960 by American Bible Society

www.xulonpress.com

Consecration

To the Lord God –

We thank you for the wisdom and knowledge you are bringing to The Church, the Body of Christ, as your great mystery is revealed. We thank you, Lord God, for those whose hearts you have prepared in advance to hear and receive this seed from the Word of God. We believe You for a great harvest, the fullness of our inheritance in Christ. May your everlasting Word cause this book to be timeless and always in season for those who encounter it. Be glorified Lord as we worship you in the manner you always intended: Spirit, Soul, and Body.

In Jesus' name,

Amen.

Dedication

To Ray,

Who are you, my beloved, who has so deeply won my heart?

You are the one the maidens sing of in the Song of Solomon. Your left arm is under my head, and your right arm embraces me. You, my love, are radiant and ruddy, outstanding among ten thousand. Your eyes are like doves by the water streams, washed in milk, mounted like jewels. Your cheeks are like beds of spice yielding perfume. Your lips are like lilies dripping with myrrh. Your arms are rods of gold. Your legs are pillars of marble set on bases of pure gold. Your appearance is like Lebanon, choice as its cedars. Your mouth is sweetness itself; you are altogether lovely. You are my lover; you are my friend. I cherish you.

Thank you for teaching me, loving me, and encouraging me to seek Him first. With long life shall He satisfy you because you have set your love upon Him! I am honored to share that life at your side. Thank you for all you poured into this project and into our lives. I love you. Mi.

Acknowledgements

There are times when a special expression of thanks and acknowledgement is appropriate. Our thanks to those mentioned here are not meant to exclude nor forget the many prayers and people who have poured the Word and the love of God into our lives for so many years, but rather an expression of our appreciation and love for specific seeds sown into this particular project.

To all our children,

> Greg, Rachelle, Kathryn, Rebecca, Billy, Renee, Christopher, Ryan
>
> (And the ones whose names we don't yet know.)

Our greatest desire for each of you is that you be woven into the tapestry of God's love, in touch with everything there is to know of God. Then you will have minds confident and at rest, focused on Christ, God's great mystery. All the richest treasures of wisdom and knowledge are embedded in that mystery, in Christ, and nowhere else.

Already, you have each in your own way gone beyond the role of children to partake as partners in this Kingdom work. We thank you for the extraordinary ways you all have expressed your belief in this project and also for the precious and significant seed some of you sowed to see it turn into sight. We pray that God will bless you and multiply your seed sown in an exceeding, abundant harvest of dreams come true.

As you walk with Him remember: There are different kinds of gifts, but the same Spirit. There are different kinds of service, but the same Lord. There are different kinds of working, but the same God works all of them *in all of you*. Do not despise nor waste your youth; but be an example of Christ, in word, in conversation, in giving, in spirit, in faith, and in purity.

We have chosen these words to you carefully. Do not neglect the gifts that are in you. Meditate upon these things; give yourselves wholly to them; in all that you do, let your lives be *evidence of His power and goodness*. Each of you has received Christ Jesus, the Master. You're deeply rooted in him. You're well constructed upon him. You know your way around the faith. Now, our beloved children do what you've been taught. Live life in abundance, to the full, until it overflows! We love you, Dad and Mom

To Mrs. Doris Ann Byrd and Miss Sandra Troutt – You, too, are partners in this Kingdom work and you have our utmost thanks for sowing your time and anointed service that it might be presented to God and the Kingdom in excellence. We ask the Lord to bless you, to fill your lives with love, and to fill your homes with rare and beautiful treasures! We love you and thank you.

To my "Freaky Friends" – I found that actually means "my friends who are so ardently devoted to God!" My sisters, you are the lifters of my hands. I love you and am forever blessed that you invited me in. Thank you for helping us birth this project in the Spirit and bring it to perfection (completeness in Him). Love, Mi

The Picture of Health®
Daily Power Plan™

Day 1 – Introduction

Ephesians 1:17-19 (New International Version)

> I keep asking that the God of our Lord Jesus Christ, the glorious Father, may give you the Spirit of wisdom and revelation, so that you may know him better.
>
> I pray also that the eyes of your heart may be enlightened in order that you may know the hope to which he has called you, the riches of his glorious inheritance in the saints, and his incomparably great power for us who believe.
>
> That power is like the working of his mighty strength…

Selah (pause and reflect)

This is a prayer that Paul prayed for those he taught in Ephesus. It is my prayer for you today and everyday. We will talk many times about wisdom and revelation in the days to come. Both work hand in hand as keys to operating in the Spirit rather than in your flesh or carnal nature. They are given freely for the asking by God to His children <u>so that we may know Him better.</u>

As you take your first "power walk" with Him today, why not ask Him to open your eyes so that you may truly see that He has called you and provided for you a rich, glorious inheritance…now in this life and the life to come. You will be learning each day in our "power walks" with God about your physical body and how to bring it under direction of the Holy Spirit. Each daily lesson from the Word will teach you about your glorious inheritance through Christ and His resurrection!

Recorded in John 4:12 (NIV), Jesus said, "I tell you the truth, anyone who has faith in me will do what I have been doing. He will do even greater things than these, because I am going to the Father." Have you thought on that scripture long enough to realize that He was speaking of things He had done while in the physical body on this natural earth? *Selah.*

Yes, through Him, resurrection power is at work to bring new life to us, **_to quicken our mortal bodies_** (Romans 8:11). That is the power that enables us to walk this out in complete victory! Praise be to God!

THE PICTURE OF HEALTH®
DAILY POWER PLAN™
Day 2

Matthew 7:24-26 (NIV)

> Therefore everyone who hears these words of mine and puts them into practice is like a wise man who built his house on the rock. The rain came down, the streams rose, and the winds blew and beat against that house; yet it did not fall, because it had its foundation on the rock. But everyone who hears these words of mine and does not put them into practice is like a foolish man who built his house on sand.

Selah (pause and reflect)

I am blessed to be able to say that my father is among Arkansas' most seasoned and respected real estate appraisers. For many years he was also a homebuilder. Before entering the healthcare field, I had the privilege of working with him and studying his profession from the inside out. We inspected many houses during my five years with him but one in particular came to mind today as I read this scripture.

We went one time to inspect a lot where new construction was beginning on a single-story starter home. We had the house plans, the plot plan, the survey, etc. As we drove up, I learned one of the greatest lessons in home building: start with a firm foundation. Here sat a crew beginning to pour foundation right on top of the ground. Now, I don't know if you know it or not, but wise builders don't do that! My dad taught me that day that one was supposed to dig down a certain depth and lay "footings" which stabilize the foundation to prevent it from shifting, settling, cracking, etc. over time. He explained that one poured on top of the ground like this one, well, was headed for trouble from day one and the ultimate cost would be uncountable over the years. (That proposed house, by the way, did not pass the first inspection!)

I think I found the description of this builder in Deuteronomy 32:28-30 (NIV), "They are a nation without sense, there is no discernment in them. If only they were wise and would understand this and discern what their end will be!" In starting that house off on the wrong footing, so to speak, he had no thought or cares for what the end would be.

The good news is that we don't have to go the way of the unwise builder. The first part of Psalm 127:1 (KJV) says, "...except the LORD build the house, they labour in vain that build it". That is the key to our scripture today.

<u>Use wisdom and let God build it!</u>

You can start by doing two things:

1) Be doers of the Word. When we put into practice the Word of God, we are like the wise man, building our house - our body, the temple of the Holy Spirit - on a solid foundation.

2) Ask for wisdom and understanding. The following verses tell us that God will give us, put into us, wisdom and understanding to do what He desires:

"Then wrought Bezaleel and Aholiab, and every wise hearted man, in whom the LORD <u>put wisdom and understanding</u> to know how

> to work all manner of work for the service of the sanctuary, according to all that the LORD had commanded." (Exodus 36:1 KJV)

The underlined emphasis is mine and there is also this verse:

> "Behold, I have done according to thy words: lo, <u>I have given thee</u> a wise and understanding heart;" (1 Kings 3:12 KJV)

Here is how you can use these passages to pray the Word into your life today:

> Father God, I thank you for your Word to me today. I thank you that you are the Builder of my house and it <u>shall not be built in vain.</u>
>
> I ask you Lord according to your Word, to put in me wisdom and understanding. Teach me so that I will know how to work all manner of work for the service of the sanctuary.
>
> Deposit your Word in me so that I know how to rightly care for my body as your dwelling place. I yield to you Lord so that, as I walk more fully in health and strength, I can greater serve your kingdom purpose.
>
> Give me, Lord, a wise and understanding heart that I can be faithful and steadfast in being a doer of your Word, putting into practice in my life all that you are teaching me.
>
> I give you all the glory Lord for the house you are building! Let all see the changes

in me and be drawn to your Light and give praise to your Holy Name! In Jesus' name, Amen.

THE PICTURE OF HEALTH®
DAILY POWER PLAN™
Day 3

1 Corinthians 6:19-20 (AMP)

> Do you not know that your body is the temple (the very sanctuary) of the Holy Spirit Who lives within you, Whom you have received [as a Gift] from God? You are not your own, You were bought with a price [purchased with a preciousness and paid for, made His own]. So then, honor God and bring glory to Him in your body.

Selah (pause and reflect)

So, here you are. Today is the day that you are starting a new program to get healthy! You are not alone.

Did you know that approximately 1/3 of all Americans have made "resolutions" this year? Those people are among the millions resolving to quit smoking, get fit, get healthy, lose weight, gain weight, etc...again.

Statistics show that 36% of those people will quit before the first month is up! And more than 1/2 (54%) will give up before six months have gone by! Why? Because all those resolutions are based on negative objectives and condemnation or guilt about some aspect of our lives. *As long as there is condemnation, there will never be freedom. There will never be victory. But...*

We have a more excellent way! A way that never fails!

Yes, beloved, if you want lasting victory, you are going to have to base your "resolution" and your motivation on something radically different. Lay aside that condemnation and guilt, which so easily besets you, and do something that never fails. What is that? **Love.**

Now watch this. The Word says *<u>love never fails.</u>* (1 Corinthians 13:8). Our scripture for today says that you were purchased with preciousness and paid for, made His own, *the temple where He abides*. If God is love (1 John 4:8), and He abides in you, then love abides in you. And… you've got it! Love never fails!

Beloved, we are going to get it this time! He is bringing us out of guilt and condemnation into His great light! We will be free from sickness and disease, beautiful, fit, and strong. We will learn to walk in love and bring glory to God in our body!

THE PICTURE OF HEALTH®
DAILY POWER PLAN™
Day 4

1 John 3:18-22 (NIV)

> Dear children, let us not love with words or tongue but with actions and in truth. This then is how we know that we belong to the truth, and how we set our hearts at rest in his presence whenever our hearts condemn us. For God is greater than our hearts, and he knows everything. Dear friends, if our hearts do not condemn us, we have confidence before God and receive from him anything we ask, because we obey his commands and do what pleases him.

Selah (pause and reflect)

Yesterday we studied that the world approaches "resolutions" from the position of guilt and condemnation...and fails. We also found that *Love,* on the other hand, *never fails.*

The age-old question is however, "Then, why are Christians still sick?" or, "Why then don't I have the healthy, strong, fit body I asked for?" I inquired of the Lord and our scripture for today was His answer to me.

To comprehend this answer, we must first look back at the scripture from yesterday. The passage asked, "Don't you know that you are the very sanctuary of the Holy Spirit?" The sanctuary is where He abides; it is the Temple, His holy dwelling place. So to fully understand the question, we must look even further back in the Word regarding the Temple, especially at the pattern given us about the care of the Temple in the Old Testament.

As I researched the Tabernacle and the Temple in the Old Testament, I found that the Lord's instruction was extremely detailed and precise to the priests about the care of His dwelling place. Because the tabernacle (and later, the Temple) was a holy dwelling place for the Spirit of the Lord, to ignore these detailed and precise instructions carried severe consequences for the priests. They died.

According to Rev 1:6 and Rev 5:10, we have been made (through Christ) the kings and priests. We, now, are the ones charged with the care of God's holy temple. Only now, the temple is not an outward building, but it is our bodies. When we fail to treat the temple as holy and consecrated, we are the ones who die. (1 Corinthians 3:16-18)

Yes, we *do* live under *grace*, and *not the law*. And, yes, *we have been redeemed from the curse* of the law of sin and death. But, when you fail to honor God in the temple (your body) you walk away from the provision that grace brings; you reject the knowledge and perish. And yes, it is by grace, through faith, that your body was redeemed and made the holy dwelling place of the Spirit of God. But, continuing to neglect the care of the temple by walking in condemnation or rebellion is a failure to receive the gift of grace that brings healing to that body!

So how are we to lay hold of the Love that never fails? How does one know if they belong to truth? Our scripture passage today gives us the keys to having confidence before God and receiving from Him anything we ask:

Love not with words or tongue (only) but *with actions and in truth.*

Are you obeying His commands? Are you doing what pleases Him? Not just in your spirit or soul, but in your body? Is the Holy Spirit leading you *in your choices* and are you *obedient to His leading* when He prompts you?

Making the choice, the commitment, to *express your love to God* through the care of temple of the Holy Spirit, in action and in truth, <u>will</u> bring about the physical victories you seek.

THE PICTURE OF HEALTH®
DAILY POWER PLAN™
Day 5

Romans 13:11-15 (AMP)

> Besides this you know what [a critical] hour this is, how it is high time now for you to wake up out of your sleep (rouse to reality). For salvation (final deliverance) is nearer to us now than when we first believed (adhered to, trusted in, and relied on Christ, the Messiah).
>
> The night is far-gone and the day is almost here. Let us then drop (fling away) the works and deeds of darkness and put on the [full] armor of light. Let us live and conduct ourselves honorably and becomingly as in the [open light of] day, not in reveling (carousing) and drunkenness, not in immorality and debauchery (sensuality and licentiousness), not in quarreling and jealousy.
>
> But clothe yourself with the Lord Jesus Christ (the Messiah), and make no provision for [indulging] the flesh [put a stop to thinking about the evil cravings of your physical nature] to [gratify its] desires (lusts).

Selah (pause and reflect)

Are you weary of destruction, illness, disease, disappointment, and dissatisfaction? Isn't it the time for you to "fling away" all that darkness and put on the *fullness* of the redemption - the *complete* victory - that Christ purchased for you: Spirit, Soul, *and Body*?

Your homework this week is to pray about making a commitment to walk in health, to possess the victory offered to you through covenant with God in Jesus Christ, to cherish and honor the physical body He gave you and redeemed for you. As you pray about making this commitment, **consider the time.**

In today's scripture from the Word of God, we are told it is high time to awake out of sleep. The Word tells us that the night is far spent. Beloved, we are closer to the Lord's Second Coming than at any other time. The Word is calling us to put on, to clothe ourselves with Christ. We are instructed to make no provision for indulging the flesh and cravings of the natural body. And even more than that, to put on, to wear, the salvation, healing, and deliverance He physically and spiritually purchased for us!

The day is at hand. Now is the time. Commit your way to the Lord and make your decision today, that this week, this year, and for all year's to come, you will open your heart and renew your mind to receive the fullness of the free gift of redemption...complete victory in your Spirit, Soul, *and Body!*

THE PICTURE OF HEALTH®
DAILY POWER PLAN™

Day 6

2 Chronicles 16:9a (NIV)

> For the eyes of the LORD range throughout the earth to strengthen those whose hearts are fully committed to him....

Selah (pause and reflect)

This first week is a special opportunity to consecrate yourself to God and fully commit your life to be used for His purpose. As we choose to make that commitment, we find in this verse a marvelous added blessing. Just as we are beginning to make changes and choices, He brings us the promise of His strength.

As you go forward in this journey, watch over your words to place His promise in action. Train yourself to use His Word aloud. Speak the Word to keep yourself on the path of righteousness. For example, instead of saying, "I can't possibly drink that much water!", speak the Word, "I can do this! I am fully committed to the Lord and His eyes are always on me to strengthen me." Or, "I can do this! I can do all things through Christ who strengthens me!" (Philippians 4:13)

Beloved, you are taking your first baby steps to divine health in Spirit, Soul, and Body! He has promised to direct those steps and He is faithful! He will watch over His Word to perform it! Never forget, not even for a moment, that you are *not* making this journey to health alone! He is leading you; His rod of correction and His staff of direction will comfort you. His eyes are upon those who are fully committed to Him to give them (you) strength!

THE PICTURE OF HEALTH®
DAILY POWER PLAN™

Day 7

Luke 12:29-31 (KJV)

> And seek not ye what ye shall eat, or what ye shall drink, neither be ye of doubtful mind. For all these things do the nations of the world seek after and your Father knoweth that ye have need of these things. But rather seek ye the kingdom of God; and all these things shall be added unto you.

Selah (pause and reflect)

Today's scripture leads me to share with you why the Lord directed us to publish The Picture of Health™ 100-day Devotional <u>first,</u> before any other books. As we sought Him for wisdom and direction, the Lord made it very clear to us:

> "Divine health is impossible to attain unless the born-again Believer seeks first to renew the mind to the Word of God."

He enabled us to see that daily, children of God seek Him for restoration in their body and for healing, then turn right around and run after the world's ways and the world's advice to try to obtain that Kingdom benefit!

Isn't that crazy? But people do it every day! Now I ask you: why would the Lord provide the benefit and then leave it up to the world – which is under the authority of your enemy Satan – to teach you how to reap that benefit? He would not. The ruler of this world doesn't want to help you walk in health! Listen, John 15:19 (NIV) says, "The world hates you."

There are thousands of "health" books that *look* like sound advice with plenty of science behind them and lots of initials after the author's name! There are hundreds of movie stars that *look* healthy, telling you about or selling you on their latest diet methods. The most common reply I hear, or actually it is an excuse, is "it *seems* to be along the same lines, basically it's the same, just a few differences, right?"

Wake up children of God! The devil has a marketing plan to snare you! The devil is a master of deception. The Bible says he comes disguised as an angel of light…but he is the enemy who comes to steal, kill, and destroy! Yes, it will look like wisdom and seem right at first. But even the devil has wisdom! (Ezekiel 28:12 and Ezekiel 28:17) Do you really think your enemy would present something so totally foreign that you would never fall for it? No! He is cunning and crafty! He is going to try to deceive you into thinking that it is acceptable to blend the world's wisdom with the Lord's wisdom.

Why? Because all Satan can do is copy (imitate) those things that he is so jealous of! He is the imposter, seeking to be your lord. His only devices remain to temp you in the lust of your eyes, the lust of your flesh, and the pride of life. Simply observed, immature or even spiritually lazy people want the appearance of godliness and health while still allowing the flesh to do what it wants to.

Face it! People want the kingdom benefit without having to change or to bring the body under submission. In a way, your actions are showing that you consider it more difficult to operate by grace and faith (by being led) than by observing the law. This "Pharisee" mindset seeks to hide behind a set of laws, keeping the very letter of it but not at all the spirit of it. In truth, when we refuse to discipline ourselves to be doers of His Word, we are only clanging cymbals and whitewashed tombs.

This is what the Lord says it, His answer to the Pharisees, in Matthew 15:7-14 (AMP)

> You pretenders (hypocrites)! Admirably and truly did Isaiah prophesy of you when he said:
>
> These people draw near Me with their mouths and honor Me with their lips, but their hearts hold off and are far away from Me. Uselessly do they worship Me, for they teach as doctrines the commands of men. And Jesus called the people to Him and said to them, Listen and grasp and comprehend this:
>
> It is not what goes into the mouth of a man that makes him unclean and defiled, but what comes out of the mouth; this makes a man unclean and defiles [him]. Then the disciples came and said to Him, Do You know that the Pharisees were displeased and offended and indignant when they heard this saying?
>
> He answered, Every plant which My heavenly Father has not planted will be torn up by the roots. Let them alone and disregard them; they are blind guides and teachers. And if a blind man leads a blind man, both will fall into a ditch.

Beloved, beneath the world's (evil) wisdom lurks deception and destruction. Paul warned the Body of Christ at Corinth about this many hundreds of years ago! The Bible records in 2 Corinthians 11:3-4 (NLT):

> But I fear that somehow you will be led away from your pure and simple devotion to Christ, just as Eve was deceived by the serpent. You seem to believe whatever anyone tells you, even if they preach about a different Jesus than the one we preach, or a different Spirit than the one you received, or a different kind of gospel than the one you believed.

The ultimate truth is you cannot seek the benefits of the Kingdom of God through the wisdom of the world! You can't even believe all those who masquerade as Christians! The enemy of your soul will take any truth and corrupt it with his ways, yet cleverly disguise it so that you buy into the lie. Don't be fooled! Further down in that same chapter of 2 Corinthians, verse 15 we are warned, "their end will be what their actions deserve".

How are you to know the difference? How are you to know what to believe? You must learn to identify the counsel of the devil and unwaveringly reject it! Jesus Christ told us how in John 14:6 (NIV) "I AM the way and the truth and the life. No one comes to the Father except through me." The Word of God is the only unchangeable truth.

You cannot avoid having to learn to *be led*.

Beloved, you cannot partake of God's provision for divine health by trying to enter the Kingdom through the world's gate. The sooner you decide to submit to the wisdom and direction of the Word, the sooner the Wisdom of God can preserve and keep you.

If you have been trying to accomplish kingdom purpose (healthy body, soul, and spirit) with worldly ways (diets, inappropriate drug use, quick fixes), you will never have lasting results. Remember, "Their end will be what their actions deserve". Your Kingdom blessings are found in the spirit not in the flesh.

Seek the kingdom of God; and all these things shall be added unto you.

The Picture of Health®
Daily Power Plan™

Day 8

2 Corinthians 12:9-10 (NIV)

> But he said to me, "My grace is sufficient for you, for my power is made perfect in weakness." Therefore I will boast all the more gladly about my weaknesses, so that Christ's power may rest on me. That is why, for Christ's sake, I delight in weaknesses, in insults, in hardships, in persecutions, in difficulties. For when I am weak, then I am strong.

Selah (pause and reflect)

Beloved, I tell you, you will want to learn this lesson early on: Real victory comes when you stop thinking you can (or have to) do this yourself, in your own strength, effort, or will power.

Already you are almost through with your first week. If you haven't had challenges yet, you can expect to encounter a few somewhere along the line. Don't despair! It is *not* a lack of faith to encounter challenges. It is only a lack of faith *if* you let them get you sidetracked!

Isaiah 40:29 encourages us that He gives strength to the weary and increases the power of the weak. When you completely surrender to the Lord and rely on Him for the power to make right choices, His power is made perfect in you.

Therefore, go forward with excitement and faith! Knowing that grace and strength will come to aid you, delight yourself in weaknesses, hardships, and difficulties. Boast when they come your way! For it is in our weakness that His power is made perfect! Stand firm! And, call upon the Name of the Lord!

THE PICTURE OF HEALTH®
DAILY POWER PLAN™

Day 9

1 Corinthians 6:12 (NIV)

> "Everything is permissible for me"–but not everything is beneficial. "Everything is permissible for me"–but I will not be mastered by anything.

Selah (pause and reflect)

"*Is this legal?*" Ah! That is the classic indication of the diet mentality at work. And then there is "I did really bad last week." Or even "I did really good last week." (Surprised at the last one?) And don't forget "*cheat*" and "*I can't have that.*"

May I just tell you plainly? **Those are all words of bondage.** Whether the goal is to lose or gain weight, lower cholesterol, or control blood sugar levels – they are all just diets – tools of the enemy to keep you in works and in bondage! The mindsets of lack and deprivation and of performance tied to reward or punishment are devices (tools) of deception from the devil (the enemy). These devices are designed to keep you in sickness and disease for as long as *you* let them!

The Word of God in John 8:32 (NIV), tells us that "you will know the **truth**, and the **truth** will set you **free**." The Word of God can make you free from the bondage of disease and diet mentalities...*forever*! But…you have to use it. You have to be a doer of the Word.

I challenge you! Next time you begin to speak words of bondage, or even think them, sternly rebuke yourself for those words or thoughts and then speak the truth instead! Renew your mind to the Word, speaking truth: "No! I will not say those words of bondage again." Or, "I can have anything I choose, anytime I choose. All things are permissible, but not all things are beneficial." And, "I refuse to be mastered by things that are not beneficial to the Temple of God!"

If you truly want to be free from disease, destruction, and dieting for the rest of your life, it is absolutely essential for you to take hold of this truth. There is power in the Word of God...be doer of the Word and that power – the anointing of God - will be actively at work in you to make you free!

THE PICTURE OF HEALTH®
DAILY POWER PLAN™
Day 10

Romans 12:1-2 (AMP)

> I appeal to you therefore, brethren, and beg of you in view of [all] the mercies of God, to make a decisive dedication of your bodies [presenting all your members and faculties] as a living sacrifice, holy (devoted, consecrated) and well pleasing to God, which is your reasonable (rational, intelligent) service and spiritual worship.
>
> Do not be conformed to this world (this age), [fashioned after and adapted to its external, superficial customs], but be transformed (changed) by the [entire] renewal of your mind [by its new ideals and its new attitude], so that you may prove [for yourselves] what is the good and acceptable and perfect will of God, even the thing which is good and acceptable and perfect [in His sight for you].

Selah (pause and reflect)

Millions of viewers tune-in to TV each week to watch one kind of reality or extreme make-over show or another, promising to dramatically change the lives of the participants forever. Thousands of dollars are spent on cosmetic procedures, diets, trainers, and clothes to "transform" them into happy, beautiful people.

Don't be fooled. Today's scripture from the Word of God reminds us that these types of changes are only external, superficial changes. Real *lasting change* comes from within.

I am *not* saying that you shouldn't buy new clothes nor have a personal trainer. No. I am not even saying that it is wrong to have cosmetic procedures. No, what I *am* saying is that the first step to permanent results in your body is the decision to truly devote or set apart *your body* to the service of God. It is an expression of your love for God. It is a sincere act of worship. It is a spiritual decision to renew your mind (your thoughts) to the Word of God so that physical health begins to blossom in your natural body *from the inside*, overflowing *to* the outside.

Our motive must be to bring glory to God!
Our methods must be learned through His Truth
and led by His Spirit.

This is why, beloved, we must stay faithful to our daily walk with Him. It is through the washing of the water of the Word of God that our minds are renewed. As we study together daily, little by little, precept upon precept, we are proving for ourselves what is the good and acceptable will of the Lord, even in regard to **our bodies.** If we persevere and faint not, we will be transformed, presenting our bodies as living sacrifices, holy, devoted, consecrated, and well pleasing to God.

THE PICTURE OF HEALTH®
DAILY POWER PLAN™
Day 11

Psalm 145:15-16 (NIV)

> The eyes of all look to you, and you give them their food at the proper time. You open your hand and satisfy the desires of every living thing.

Selah (pause and reflect)

Are your old habits and choices trying to interrupt your plans for success? Are you feeling the temptation to first say the wrong thing and then do the wrong thing? If so, you may be asking, "How do I keep on the right path? How do I remain steadfast in my commitment? How do I stay excited and in faith?"

Here's your answer: Put the Word of God in front of your eyes, in your ears, down in your heart, and speak it out your mouth!

When you sense that you are about to whine or complain, correct yourself and apply the Word of Truth instead. These daily "power walks" with God are not just for us to read. Their purpose is to exercise our faith and heal our bodies! We are to go beyond just reading. We are to act upon them each day!

For example, you should take today's verse and commit to your heart this truth: "The Lord gives me food at the proper time and God Himself opens His hand and satisfies me!" Then when you are tempted, the truth can speak out,

"I can *easily* choose not to have that extra sugar right now (or caffeine or whatever) because I am **well satisfied** by the Lord's hand. He gives me all things at the proper time!"

Now don't be shy and lose your victory! Learn to believe and speak the Word out loud. Make choices to edify (build up) yourself in health. Rather than give into the desires of the carnal flesh, lay hold of the truth of the Word of God. It is written that the Word does not return void but accomplishes that for which He sent it.

It will work if you do it by faith!

THE PICTURE OF HEALTH®
DAILY POWER PLAN™
Day 12

Jude 1:24-25 (NIV)

To him who is able to keep you from falling and to present you before his glorious presence without fault and with great joy– [25]to the only God our Savior be glory, majesty, power and authority, through Jesus Christ our Lord, before all ages, now and forevermore! Amen.

Selah (pause and reflect)

Have you realized it? You are on a journey like none you have ever taken. We, the Children of Grace, are setting ourselves apart for these 100 days to renew our minds to the Word of God. Whether you know it yet or not, we are making changes in our Spirit and Soul (mind, will, and emotions) that will affect our lives, including our physical bodies, for all our days.

What I'd like you to see today is that this entire path will not only bring change to our bodies, but to every area of our lives if we let it. You could see this as a type of fast – or actually "feast" is a more appropriate word. We are feasting on the Word of *God with purpose.* And that purpose is not to move God…but *to move us*, to draw nearer to God so that His will becomes our desire, Spirit, Soul, and Body.

The Lord recently showed it to me this way: everything of the Kingdom of God magnifies God, glorifies God, and draws you and others to God. If whatever you are doing draws yours focus to you, it is not of God. For example, diets draw one's focus to the dieter and his or her actions or performance. In contrast, the mission of The Picture of Health Series™ is to draw your focus to God and the Kingdom of God. That is why this 100-day devotional was the first book He released us to publish (even though we have several others in writing at this time.) The Lord impressed on our hearts that this had to be *first*, reminding us of Matthew 6:33, (NIV) "But seek first his kingdom and his righteousness, and all these things will be given to you as well." In fact, that whole chapter of Matthew addresses this very mindset, even in regard to food and drink.

Why do I share this with you today? I share it today because by now you are several days into your 100-day walk with God, exercising your faith and healing your body. I felt led by the Holy Spirit to encourage you and challenge you to press in! In The Picture of Health™ Series, you learn through the light of love about the power that works in you to produce health, fullness of joy and the fruits of abiding in the Kingdom blessing.

These 100 days should draw you to Him and should daily magnify His power at work in us to glorify Him in this temple! We should daily become less self-conscious and more God-conscious. As we do, we better understand our verse for today, which tells us that it is He who is able to keep us from falling. It is He who is able to present you before his glorious presence without fault and with great joy.

The Picture of Health® Daily Power Plan™
Day 13

John 6:51 (KJV)

> I am the living bread which came down from heaven: if any man eat of this bread, he shall live for ever: and the bread that I will give is my flesh, which I will give for the life of the world.

Selah (pause and reflect)

One day in class, a patient, Nancy, asked me, "What if you don't crave sweets or breads, you just *like* them?" "Well," I replied, "could you leave them off completely – without any difficulty - for thirty days if you chose to do so?"

Most people could *not* truthfully answer "yes" to that question. More often than not, especially if you have consumed generous amounts of grains or sweets for quite sometime, you would find yourself quite surprised at the intensity of the withdrawal. Cravings, shakiness, irritability, moodiness, and lack of energy are all withdrawal symptoms. These can come as a result of physical sources such as parasites, yeast, or sugar addictions, but can also come from the mental habit or emotional eating pattern. The truth is millions of people are in bondage in this area just like any other addiction.

The American Heritage® Dictionary defines addiction as a "compulsive physiological and psychological need for a habit-forming substance" but it also defines addiction as **"the condition of being habitually or compulsively** *occupied with or involved in something."* Beloved, when you have truly made Jesus Christ the Lord of your life the only thing that we should be habitually or compulsively occupied with or involved in is our relationship with the Him!

Are food, drink, size, shape, weight, sickness and disease, compulsively occupying your every day? If that is true for you, it is time to get free! This week you can join the others participating in The Picture of Health® wellness classes and begin to bring your life back in balance.

Beloved, there are *times* for feasting. But the Bible cautions us in Proverbs 23 about giving in to gluttony (defined as "to eat in excess, especially when habitual"). Frequent indulgences in sugars and grains rob us of health and make us "poor". But…frequent indulgences in the *Living Bread* build health and give life!

If your life has been out of balance, if you can't seem to put down the indulgences of the flesh, it is time cease from your feasting and to begin fasting, like we spoke of yesterday. Repent for turning to food, drink, sickness, approval, or any other addiction to find your identity. Ask the Lord to strengthen you as you choose to lay aside that which takes His place as the object of love in your life. Then, write your scriptures out on index cards and keep them with you. Look at them or read them aloud anytime you struggle. Instead of feeding the flesh and unholy addictions, feed the desire to partake of the bread of life!

As you walk in victory with the Lord today, let the confession of your mouth be "I am well satisfied by the hand of God and eating richly on the living bread that gives me life!"

THE PICTURE OF HEALTH®
DAILY POWER PLAN™
Day 14

Titus 2:11-12 (NLT)

> For the grace of God has been revealed, bringing salvation to all people. And we are instructed to turn from godless living and sinful pleasures. We should live in this evil world with self-control, right conduct, and devotion to God,

Selah (pause and reflect):

Take a deep breath in. Can you smell the rich aroma of the Bread of Life? What? You don't smell anything? Don't you have your index card in your pocket to partake of that bread at any time? Didn't you read with me yesterday?

Wait a minute. Don't tell me you are still holding on to something other than the Lord? Are you? Are you still feeding the flesh because you are "just not there yet"? Or perhaps you have "technically" abstained from eating sweets and breads, but are still *longing* in your heart for it and counting the days until you can feast on them again? If that is you, I have a *strong* word for you today, in love.

Beloved, this is not just about bread or cookies or weight or blood sugar!

It is about devotion and faith.

Look at Abraham. Years ago, God moved on Abraham's heart much like I believe He is moving on the hearts of His children in this hour. The Lord called Abraham to lay upon the altar the most precious object of his affection – his son Isaac – to offer him up, to release him to God. In response to that beckoning, Abraham brought faith. He did not grieve and try to hold on. Why? How could he do such a difficult thing without a struggle? Because <u>he trusted God.</u> Genesis 22:14 (NIV) says, "So Abraham called that place The LORD Will Provide. And to this day it is said, 'On the mountain of the LORD it will be provided.'"

OK. So maybe you are thinking, 'that was Abraham's <u>son,</u> not breads, sweets, junk food, or sugar.' But isn't it still about the object of your affection? How much easier should it be to lay natural things (breads, sweets, junk food, or sugar) on that altar than one of our children or loved ones! Right, it should be! *Then why haven't you?*

Food, drink, or the sickness identity has become *your* loved one.

I am sorry if that realization pierces deep for some of you. Perhaps you are even shedding tears at this moment. Go ahead…let the love of God heal you. Let Him become the one you love.

I know that for many of you, surrender and freedom have been a long time in coming. But beloved, today is the day of deliverance for you who will receive it! Today it is my desire, like the Lord's desire, to pierce through the darkness and bring you the Light. Whatever it is that you love more than God – that is what is required of you on the altar today.

Do not be afraid to let go of whatever it is you love.

Nothing compares to the riches we gain in Christ.

God sacrificed His only Son, Jesus Christ, so that you could be free from sin, <u>and its wages of death,</u> both in this life and the eternal life to come. He is the Bread of Life! He is our provider! He is Jehovah Jireh! He is the one who sees ahead and provides for our redemption. He is the Lord Jehovah who supplies what you need – by His grace - when you place all things precious to you on the altar and receive His sacrifice in place of yours. He will provide!

It is not difficult. It doesn't take a lot of time. Just simply ask Him – right now - for His grace that will strengthen you to turn away from that which lasts only for the moment, sinful pleasures that leave destruction in their wake.

Today is your day of freedom. As you choose to make Him truly the Lord of *all* your life - spirit, soul, *and body* - He will supply all your needs. You will never lack. You will never come short. As you <u>act</u> in devotion to Him, He will bless you beyond what you can ask, think, or even imagine!

THE PICTURE OF HEALTH®
DAILY POWER PLAN™
Day 15

2 Corinthians 3:17 (AMP)

> Now the Lord is the Spirit, and where the Spirit of the Lord is, there is liberty (emancipation from bondage, freedom).

Selah (pause and reflect)

F. F. Bosworth said, "Faith begins where the will of God is known." Our scripture focus today very plainly shows us that bondage is not God's will for our lives:

"Where the Spirit of the Lord is, there is freedom."

Examine your life. Is legalism part of your upbringing or heritage? Are guilt, frustration and fear over disease, or even over your appearance, part of your life? If the answer is yes in any measure, then you are in bondage.

It is the Lord's greatest desire that you be free from bondage, death, and destruction. Look at these scriptures:

> The Spirit of the Lord God is upon me, because the Lord has anointed and qualified me to preach the Gospel of good tidings to the meek, the poor, and afflicted; He has sent me to bind up and heal the brokenhearted, to proclaim liberty to the [physical and spiritual] captives and the opening of the prison and of the eyes to those who are bound (Isaiah 61:1 AMP)

And:

> And Jesus replied to them, Go and report to John what you hear and see: The blind receive their sight and the lame walk, lepers are cleansed (by healing) and the deaf hear, the dead are raised up and the poor have good news (the Gospel) preached to them. And blessed (happy, fortunate, and to be envied) is he who takes no offense at Me and finds no cause for stumbling in or through Me and is not hindered from seeing the Truth. (Matthew 11:4-6 AMP)

You can see even more as you read Luke 4:18-19 and Luke 7:22. His message is clear: God wants you whole, healed, saved, delivered, and set free from *all* bondage! This is the very purpose for which He sent his Son Jesus Christ to die for you and me.

As you spend some time with the Lord this week, *press in* to the Word and seek out this truth - not as religion...but as the truth that will make you (permanently, eternally) free! Realize that your physical body is part of His redemption (Galatians 3:13) and determine to walk in the freedom, the divine health, He purchased for you!

THE PICTURE OF HEALTH®
DAILY POWER PLAN™
Day 16

Romans 15:13 (KJV)

> Now the God of hope fill you with all joy and peace in believing, that ye may abound in hope, through the power of the Holy Ghost.

Selah (pause and reflect)

Today is a day of refreshing. Instead of a longer devotional time today, let's meditate (think on, focus with purpose, continually come back to the thought) on being filled with joy and peace so that we can overflow with hope for these coming days.

It isn't always easy to make life changes. But, according to Nehemiah 8:10, we are not to sorrow, for the joy of the Lord is our strength. So, today I say to you,

"Receive fresh courage! The power of the Holy Spirit is daily filling us with the joy of the Lord. Abide, dwell in, stay in, *and live* in the secret place of the Most High. His joy will strengthen you and bring you peace for the journey."

THE PICTURE OF HEALTH®
DAILY POWER PLAN™
Day 17

1 Timothy 4:1-5 (NIV) *(Note: italics mine)*

> The Spirit clearly says that in later times some will abandon the faith and follow deceiving spirits and things taught by demons. Such teachings come through hypocritical liars, whose consciences have been seared as with a hot iron. They forbid people to marry and *order them to abstain from certain foods, which God created to be received with thanksgiving by those who believe and who know the truth. For everything God created is good, and nothing is to be rejected if it is received with thanksgiving, because it is consecrated by the word of God and prayer.*

Selah (pause and reflect)

Should we eat meat or not? Should we eat only raw foods? Can we have cooked foods? Was Jesus a vegetarian? These are all questions Christians are asking after reading one or more of the dozens of books telling you how a Christian "should" eat. With so many conflicting bits of advice, many Christians have been left in confusion.

Let's address that from the Word. 1 Corinthians 14:33 says that God is not the author of confusion, but of peace. Confusion should be our first clue that they are on the wrong path. Look again at today's scripture passage. Everything God created is good and nothing is to be rejected if it is received with thanksgiving. That is not confusing._

I believe that is when my friend Bob contributed to class, "So, we can eat and drink anything and everything we want and still be healthy as long as we are thankful for it!" Not exactly, Bob. Nice try though. You see it is man who has carried his liberty to the extreme and has taken advantage of grace. People have become rebellious, gluttonous and greedy, even to their own destruction.

And, perhaps worse than that, in an attempt to bring the body of Christ back to health, many Bible teachers and even doctors have gone in the "opposite ditch". Many today try to convince people that they must return to the eating instructions given by the Lord in various parts of the Old Testament if they want the blessing of (New Testament) health.

Consider this: without light, people return to what they view as the safety of the law - just like the Israelites who thought to return to the slavery of Egypt preferable to their time in the desert!

Some have insisted that the Bible teaches us to be vegetarians or raw food consumers only. Some lean toward eating from the traditional foods of the Mediterranean culture. Still others believe we are to eat a diet high in protein, called a Paleolithic diet. (And then of course, there is low fat, which isn't even in the Bible.) Three main problems arise from all of these teachings. First, we are not under the law. We are under grace. Second, compromise and inconsistency are inevitable because we cannot keep the entire law. And, finally, the focus is on food, not on God and the expression of our love for Him or the desire to glorify him in our choices and in our bodies!

I imagine these people are well meaning in their attempts to bring help to the body of Christ. However, diets and laws, legalism, is <u>not</u> the way to victory. Our scripture for today from the Word of God cautions us about diets and rigid eating plans - even going so far as to tell us they are from demons and hypocritical liars! God wants you to see that by His great provision, we have been set free from the law - redeemed from its burden and its curse by Christ.

Here, look at this scripture in Romans 3:28-31 (NLT): *(italics mine)*

> So we are made right with God through faith and not by obeying the law. After all, God is not the God of the Jews only, is he? Isn't he also the God of the Gentiles? Of course he is. There is only one God, and there is only one way of being accepted by him. *He makes people right with himself only by faith, whether they are Jews or Gentiles. Well then, if we emphasize faith, does this mean that we can forget about the law? Of course not! In fact, only when we have faith do we truly fulfill the law.*

It is <u>by faith</u> that we break free the bondage of food and drink. It is <u>by faith</u> that we learn to give thanks to the Lord for both, given at the proper time from God, in balance and with grace. By the same grace with faith, if the Lord, through the leading of the Holy Spirit, directs you to exclude foods that are not beneficial or to limit certain things that have mastered you in the past, do so quickly! And purpose to do it without rebellion or condemnation! Willingly and obediently bring your flesh under submission of your spirit!

Remember, in freedom, we have chosen to re-build the temple to glorify God. It is by faith and through your devotion to Him that you will truly discover that you are free from diets forever!

THE PICTURE OF HEALTH®
DAILY POWER PLAN™
Day 18

Hebrews 13:9 (AMP)

> Do not be carried about by different and varied and alien teachings; for it is good for the heart to be established and ennobled and strengthened by means of grace (God's favor and spiritual blessing) and not [to be devoted to] foods [rules of diet and ritualistic meals], which bring no [spiritual] benefit or profit to those who observe them.

Hebrews 13:9 (NLT)

> So do not be attracted by strange, new ideas. Your spiritual strength comes from God's special favor, not from ceremonial rules about food, which don't help those who follow them.

Selah (pause and reflect)

Look at the world. There are diets promising to prevent disease, diets for weight loss, diets for weight gain, and diets for diabetics. If you can name it, there is a diet for it. The thing is, none of them are working! Our society is in worse shape with the greatest number of eating disorders, obesity, diabetes, and all disease, than there has ever been recorded. People are on restricted diets for heart disease... yet still dying of it. People are on diets to lose weight...yet still obese and getting heavier every year. There are children on diets for allergies, asthma, learning and behavior difficulties...yet the epidemic worsens yearly. *Doesn't the evidence speak for itself?* The diet approach to any disease brings no profit to those who follow it!

<u>*Your goals in the physical body can only be established by His strength and grace.*</u>

Friends, I can't "sugar coat it" (**pun** intended): It's time to separate yourself from the world and be obedient to the Word of God. Let today's scripture from the Word of God really settle deep down in your spirit. Read it a few times out loud, letting it speak to your heart. Faith comes by hearing the Word of God.

His strength and grace is there for you. Decide today that you will not be devoted to rules of diets and determine that your strength will come from Him. And, when people begin to notice how healthy you are becoming, give God the glory! Just tell them, "It's God's special favor working in me!"

THE PICTURE OF HEALTH®
DAILY POWER PLAN™
Day 19

Galatians 5:16 (NIV)

> So I say, live by the Spirit, and you will not gratify the desires of the sinful nature.

Galatians 5:16 (The Message)

> My counsel is this: Live freely, animated and motivated by God's Spirit. Then you won't feed the compulsions of selfishness.

Selah (pause and reflect)

The Word of God brings light, understanding, and revelation as to what or who is leading us or controlling us. Our scripture today teaches us that if you are living by the Spirit of God (being Spirit-led) you will *not* satisfy the lusts or desires of the flesh. (That's your carnal sin-nature, including your physical body.)

So…if we *are* gratifying the lusts, pleasure of the flesh, the conclusion must be that the Spirit of God is not the one who is leading us! But we can change that!

Notice that The Message translation says, "…you won't feed the compulsions of selfishness". That is our clue. Examine your thoughts and actions. Do compulsions or cravings lead you? If the answer is yes, then the flesh is ruling, or mastering, you!

Beloved, we have already determined in previous days that according to the Word of God, we will not be mastered by anything except The Master, Jesus Christ! Now it is time that we act on the Word and bring the flesh under submission to the Spirit.

Just as a child learns from verbal instruction and consistency, so can your body! Instruct your flesh with your words. Answer your cravings with strong, bold statements of faith like, "No! I am no longer going to feed the compulsions of selfishness and the lusts of my flesh." Or, "I am *not* going to give in to that! I have strength and grace from God." And, my favorite, "Shut up flesh. I do not live by your cravings any more! I live fully consecrated unto God, called and chosen for His purpose!"

THE PICTURE OF HEALTH®
DAILY POWER PLAN™
Day 20

Romans 8:12-14 (NIV)

> Therefore, brothers, we have an obligation–but it is not to the sinful nature, to live according to it. For if you live according to the sinful nature, you will die; but if by the Spirit you put to death the misdeeds of the body, you will live, because those who are led by the Spirit of God are sons of God.

<u>Selah (pause and reflect)</u>

Many people read through today's scriptures and see only a spiritual message. I challenge you to read it again. "…but if by the Spirit you put to death the misdeeds of the body…" No matter how many times you read that, there is no denying that these scriptures from the Word speak directly about the results of our choices in the body.

This is the real meat of the Word folks. Paul is laying it out very plainly so that we can't possibly miss it: We have an *obligation* to the mercy and grace that has been shown to us by God. We see this again in Romans 12:1, where the Word urges us "in view of God's mercy, <u>to offer your bodies</u> as living sacrifices, holy and pleasing to God—this is your spiritual act of worship."

Beloved, this health journey is not merely for us. If you are making changes just so you can look better or even feel better, you do not yet fully understand the *power of purpose.* In truth, our greatest desire should be to glorify Him and bring the gospel (good news) to the nations!

Now listen. Hear me. That doesn't mean the body is not important. It is. Our obligation doesn't exclude the body…it <u>includes</u> it! Why else did Christ have to come in the flesh to accomplish the propitiation (payment) for our sins? Why else would he have been whipped in the flesh so that by His stripes we might be healed? Why else did He have to be bruised in the body for our iniquities (continuing sins committed in spirit, soul, and body)? These are all things that happened in the natural to accomplish a spiritual purpose!

So, yes! Our redemption by grace and our obligation to that grace includes the body. But it is in our glorifying Him that He has provided the way for us to have that victory! Results in our physical bodies – looking good and living healthy - are directly related to our heart being open to receive from Him and fulfill our purpose in Him.

The only way to lasting health is through relationship with Jesus Christ, including our praise and worship of Him and <u>our obedience to His *every* direction</u> – in our spirit, soul <u>and body</u>!

If you have missed the mark in this area, repent and use these daily walks with Him to renew your mind. Resolve to <u>stop separating</u> your spiritual walk from <u>the actions</u> of your natural body. Learn instead to <u>apply your spiritual walk in governing the actions</u> of the natural body.

THE PICTURE OF HEALTH®
DAILY POWER PLAN™
Day 21

Matthew 11:28-30 (The Message)

> Are you tired? Worn out? Burned out on religion? Come to me. Get away with me and you'll recover your life. I'll show you how to take a real rest. Walk with me and work with me—watch how I do it. Learn the unforced rhythms of grace. I won't lay anything heavy or ill-fitting on you. Keep company with me and you'll learn to live freely and lightly.

Selah (pause and reflect)

Have you noticed the theme in our walks this week? Every verse we have studied has spoken to our hearts about God's message to us, in our bodies, to live free, consecrated unto God through prayer and the Word, strengthened by grace, living by His Spirit, giving life to the mortal body.

These scriptures bring us the light of revelation that we are not only saved by His grace to spend eternity with Him, but He also has provided life, health, and strength *for today in this physical body!* Today's scripture adds to us rest for our weary soul (our mind, will, and emotions).

So, why are so many of us still struggling? Why doesn't every Christian have health and victory in the body *and* rest in their mind? Well, perhaps some do not yet know the Word of God provides that for them. Others simply have not acknowledged the importance God's Word puts on the care of the temple and the obligation to the grace given us. Still others, and probably most, have side-stepped and remained purposely blind to the issue in order to avoid the choices it takes to bring the flesh under submission of the Spirit. (Ouch! I guess the last one smarts a bit?)

Most of our modern societies don't care much for the word *"submission"*. Somewhere along the road, man (and woman) has made "submission" into an ugly image of *"oppression"*. But, Beloved, that is the world's view of it because that is the way the world dominates - with fear and control.

Oppression subtracts from your worth
and brings bondage.

That very bondage is <u>why it seems hard</u> for you to make right choices! As long as you are operating in the flesh, the carnal nature, the world's system, it will be hard!

But, Glory to God! That is not true in the kingdom of God. You see the kingdom of God operates on His Love and authority.

True submission in love and to brings greater fulfillment
and freedom.

For example, when a true Christian husband and wife choose to willingly submit themselves one to another, the wife gains a cherished position, on a pedestal, adored as Christ adores the Church, and the husband gains a place of leadership and true honor, respected by all who know him.

This dynamic principle also holds true when we, as children of God, willingly offer ourselves, our bodies, as a living sacrifice to the Lord as His dwelling place. Our act of *joyful submission* engages the power of heaven to bring freedom and victory. The Lord says His way is easy, His yoke is light! (Mat 11:30 KJV)

To finally experience complete freedom from that heavy-laden yoke of disease, diets, and defeat, you must *feed* on today's scripture from the Word.

As you complete your quiet time with the Lord today, your company with God will teach you to live freely and lightly. Say the passage aloud and *really listen* to His voice. The translation used from *The Message* *beautifully* expresses His heartfelt desire for you. As you meditate on the Word, you will hear His exquisite love inviting you to "*learn the unforced rhythms of grace*".

He promises you, beloved, if you walk with Him, you will recover your life.

The Picture of Health®
Daily Power Plan™
Day 22

Deuteronomy 7:22 (NIV)

> The LORD your God will drive out those nations before you, little by little. You will not be allowed to eliminate them all at once, or the wild animals will multiply around you.

Selah (pause and reflect)

Ever feel like your old habits and cravings are about to take over? The Lord knows that. And He has a plan that will help you!

When the children of God first spied out the Promised Land, all but two of the spies returned with bad reports. They were afraid and cried that there were beasts and giants who made them feel like grasshoppers in comparison. Looking at the task all at once, they lost courage to even begin to enter the land.

That's how it is with taking back what He has promised and given you: *health.* You can't do this overnight or all the changes at once! The wisdom of God says you must seek to drive out the nations (disease, diets, and the world's system of thinking and doing) little by little. Otherwise, the wild beasts (all your old choices and habits and fleshly desires) will multiply around you!

The only ones who entered the Promised Land were the ones who were patient and had faith in God's ability to deliver what He had promised! The ones who were too afraid of the giants had neither patience nor faith. Those who did not believe in God's strength sabotaged their own great future and died in the wilderness.

Praise God! You *are not* of them who don't believe! *You have faith!* Verse 21 of Deuteronomy 7 says, "Do not be terrified by them, for the LORD your God, who is among you, is a great and awesome God." So don't get discouraged if you don't see it happen overnight!

Little by little He will drive out the nations before you!

Together, we will take the land!

THE PICTURE OF HEALTH®
DAILY POWER PLAN™
Day 23

Matthew 23:25-27 (NLT)

> How terrible it will be for you teachers of religious law and you Pharisees. Hypocrites! You are so careful to clean the outside of the cup and the dish, but inside you are filthy—full of greed and self-indulgence! Blind Pharisees! First wash the inside of the cup, and then the outside will become clean, too.
>
> How terrible it will be for you teachers of religious law and you Pharisees. Hypocrites! You are like whitewashed tombs—beautiful on the outside but filled on the inside with dead people's bones and all sorts of impurity.

Selah (pause and reflect):

In *The Picture of Health®* classes, students learn that the primary causes of disease and dysfunction are insufficiency, trauma, and toxicity. Today, I'd like us to look at that topic of toxicity or "uncleanness" from a biblical perspective.

To be unclean in the Bible is to be diseased, cursed. A more thorough study of the Word on this shows us that this uncleanness can be found in your spirit, soul, *or* body. The passage above from Matthew 23 addresses a group of hypocrites not unlike some are today. These people live a life of pretend. They pretend to love God and have the appearance of walking a spiritual life. Their actions, however, show otherwise.

Real cleanness, life and health, comes from the inside - this applies to the spirit and soul, as well as the body and overflows to the outside. It is *not* the other way around. The Pharisees evidently looked well from the outside, physically and spiritually obeying all the rules. But the Lord saw uncleanness inside, both in their souls (greed and pride in their religious actions) and in their bodies (self-indulgence and dead men's bones).

We can glean wisdom from these examples. Ask yourself, "What has one achieved if your 'talk' is right but your walk is wrong?" I mean, suppose you put on a great Christian image to those around you, but the words you speak never have an effect, for example, on the way you treat your physical body, the temple of God and His great gift to you? Or, ask yourself, "If you achieve a certain look on the outside (whitewashed and pretty), but are filled with disease on the inside, what have you accomplished?" The Word says "dead men's bones".

Our life's purpose is to bring God glory and accomplish that for which we are created. Matthew 5:14 (NLT) says, "You are the light of the world—like a city on a mountain, glowing in the night for all to see." Beloved, I encourage you today to choose – make a decisive act - not to have any part in *dead men's bones* ever again! As He leads us, we will learn to first clean the inside (spirit, soul, *and body*) and the outside will be clean!

THE PICTURE OF HEALTH®
DAILY POWER PLAN™
Day 24

Matthew 25:10 (NLT)

> But while they were gone to buy oil, the bridegroom came, and those who were ready went in with him to the marriage feast, and the door was locked.

Matthew 25:13 (NIV)

> Therefore keep watch, because you do not know the day or the hour.

Selah (pause and reflect):

Don't you just love weddings? I just marvel at how brides always seem to glow with that special radiance! Do you know what I mean? There is that special light and that certain sparkle. There is a glow from the holy passion that is awakening within her, God's anointed gift meant only for her beloved. By the wedding day, she has carefully prepared herself to be presented to him, without spot or wrinkle. It is her indication to her beloved that she cherishes his proposal and that she joyfully awaits this holy union sanctified and blessed by God. What a beautiful beginning to a lifetime of love!

Our scripture today from the Word of God takes a look at the preparations for the wedding feast. In this text, there were maidens, virgins, who *by faith* prepared. Their lamps glowed, ready, with extra oil to spare, cherishing the invitation. And then there were others who did not, taking the invitation lightly, thinking they had all the time to do as they wished. When the bridegroom came, the ones who were prepared went with him into the wedding feast. The virgins who took things for granted suddenly found themselves unprepared and the door was shut without them!

What is this scripture speaking to us? We are cautioned to be watchful because we don't know how much time we have. The bridegroom is warning us, "Don't let the door shut with you on the outside. It is time to trim your wicks and fill the lamps with oil!"

But, what does that mean? It means <u>value the gift of life, health, and deliverance.</u>

In practical terms, it means stop being selfish and self-indulgent while your oil - your health - dwindles away! If you use it all up on yourself, you won't have any left for His plans.

Beloved, I encourage you…don't waste one more precious day! He redeemed our health now so that His purpose in us might be fulfilled. The Word is truth. This life is but a vapor. If we idly waste away the time, the door will shut on this life and *our* opportunity for His great purpose will be gone. Be diligent and prepared. <u>Attend to your lamp.</u>

THE PICTURE OF HEALTH®
DAILY POWER PLAN™
Day 25

1 Peter 1:13 (NIV)

> Therefore, prepare your minds for action; be self-controlled; set your hope fully on the grace to be given you when Jesus Christ is revealed.

Selah (pause and reflect):

Attend your lamp. Isn't that another way of saying, "prepare"? This seems to be the message of the hour all over the Kingdom of God. *Why?* **Faith prepares**.

If you believe it is God's will for you to be healthy and honor Him in the temple, then *by faith*, you must prepare, and in this case, the Word says **prepare your minds** *for action*! Hebrews Chapter 11 is *filled* with people whom God singled out for mention to all generations <u>because they each prepared</u> "by faith" *for action*.

So, what are you doing to prepare *by faith* for your new healthy body?

The scripture verse in 1 Peter tells us two things we can begin doing: be self-controlled and set our hope on God's grace. What happens when you hope for something? You prepare for it! Think about an expectant couple, an eager child before a special celebration, or a bride-to-be before her wedding day. Do any of these wait for the moment to arrive before doing anything? Not if they are excited and filled with hope about it!

The Bible says that we are the Bride of Christ! I sense that even after our "walk" yesterday, some of you are still not preparing yourselves for the wedding day, the day when He will take you to Himself without spot or blemish.

Perhaps you delay, thinking as many do that HE has to do that for us...make us without spot or blemish.

The truth is...*He has*. He *has* supplied the price that was paid for my redemption. He *has* taken the stripes and pain in His own body for my healing. He *has* taken upon Him all the oppression from the enemy so that I am delivered from darkness into light. *HE HAS*.

If your life and body don't reflect that, then the question remains, have you *received* what He has provided? Have you taken it into yourself and do you honor it by treating the temple He redeemed as holy?

We looked yesterday at the parable of the ten virgins. Today in Matthew 22:1-14, Jesus tells us of the parable of the wedding banquet. Many who were *invited* were too busy and selfish or self-absorbed to come. So the master *chose* others. Jesus' parable tells of a guest who did not bother to dress for the wedding and perished because of it. Some hold that it was the custom to provide clothes for those attending if they had none and thus the guest had no excuse for the disrespectful appearance. Others believe the guest may have just arrived in soiled garments rather than valuing the invitation and carefully preparing. In either instance, it was an outrageous insult to the gracious invitation of the master. The scripture tells us that the guest was thrown out into the darkness!

The wedding feast approaches. Now is the time for His chosen bride to ready herself, to clothe herself in the splendor that He provides for us. Set your hope on His grace and, by faith, ready yourself (prepare) in the manner worthy of the invitation!

> "...For many are invited, but few are chosen."
> (Matthew 22:14 NIV)

THE PICTURE OF HEALTH®
DAILY POWER PLAN™
Day 26

Galatians 1:10 (NIV)

> Am I now trying to win the approval of men, or of God? Or am I trying to please men? If I were still trying to please men, I would not be a servant of Christ.

Selah (pause and reflect)

Are you addicted to approval? Have you stopped to ask yourself, "What is my motivation for wanting change in the physical body?" Is it your appearance, your weight, someone's attention or approval, a boost to your self-esteem? The truth is that all of those reasons are usually fear-based, people-pleasing reasons and reactions of the flesh.

Those things can be important, but only when the Holy Spirit motivates us and the purpose of our actions is to line up with the Word of God. When we seek the approval of others and use this to determine our actions, we are operating not by the Spirit, but by the flesh. Romans 8:8 (KJV) tells us that they that are in the flesh cannot please God.

Approval addiction, competition, appearances, and poor self-esteem fuel the multi-*billion* dollar diet, drug, and beauty industry each year! And still, 60% of Americans are clinically obese, 60% have or will soon have diabetes, and millions more have cancer, heart disease, eating disorders, and other diseases.

This is not the way for a child of God to live! We are joint heirs with Christ, chosen to rule and reign! We have the gospel of the Kingdom of God, the good news that we are saved, healed, and delivered from every curse! If you have been in bondage to approval addiction, it is high time to determine that the Word of God is your lamp and let it light the way to freedom!

Don't be discouraged if it takes a little time to regain your health. Refuse to listen to what others say about you unless their words agree with His Word. Victory in your physical body only comes when we reject the works of the flesh and the opinions of men. Then we can approach the throne of God's mercy and grace by faith!

> But without faith it is impossible to please him: for he that cometh to God must believe that he is, and that he is a rewarder of them that diligently seek him. Hebrews 11:6 (KJV)

THE PICTURE OF HEALTH®
DAILY POWER PLAN™
Day 27

Luke 15:17 (NIV)

> When he came to his senses, he said, 'How many of my father's hired men have food to spare, and here I am starving to death!'

<u>Selah (pause and reflect)</u>

Ever notice? It is the nature of the carnal man to want to do it our own way and follow the way of the world. Unfortunately, it usually lands us exactly where this young man found himself…in a smelly, ugly, mess! The Word tells us that when he "came to himself" or "came to his senses", he had a great revelation: His father's way was better after all!

As you read the entire text in Luke 15, you will discover that the son humbly repented and sought the father's forgiveness. Upon seeing the son had returned, the father rushed to his side, robed him with fine clothes, and welcomed him with a grand feast!

That is exactly how your Heavenly Father is!

He is there waiting and watching for you and ready to fully restore you. Isn't this the time to stop doing it your way and the world's way, ending up in frustration, disease, and despair? With one simple, sincere statement of repentance, you can receive God's forgiveness and begin walking again in His excellent plan for your life!

Today, beloved, come to your senses and come home to your Father's arms!

> For I know the plans I have for you…plans to prosper you and not to harm you, plans to give you hope and a future. Jeremiah 29:11 (NIV)

THE PICTURE OF HEALTH®
DAILY POWER PLAN™
Day 28

Philippians 3:3 (NIV)

> For it is we who are the circumcision, we who worship by the Spirit of God, who glory in Christ Jesus, and who put no confidence in the flesh.

Selah (pause and reflect)

As you spend your quiet time with the Lord today, reflect on the emphasis of this scripture: It is about God…not you. Beloved, it is time to settle this issue of works once and for all. It is time to get your mind off of you and on El Shaddai – God who is more than enough!

When we fix our eyes on Him our perspective changes. We worship by the Spirit of God. We glory in Christ. We <u>don't</u> put our confidence in *our* flesh. There isn't one person on earth that hasn't experienced the limitations of our earthly abilities! It has to be the height of ignorance to think we can do anything worth doing without Him. But with Him! Oh! My friends, there is a glorious difference! He tells us how: *through* our praise and worship of the Most High God!

Place yourself in a new level of success today. Realize the power of His might at work in you and place your trust in Christ. It is only His ability that can see you through this to victory! You do your part by staying faithful to your decision to be willing and obedient; to follow what His Word directs you to do. As you do, He promises that you shall eat the good of the land!

THE PICTURE OF HEALTH®
DAILY POWER PLAN™
Day 29

Nehemiah 8:10 (The Message)

> He continued, "Go home and prepare a feast, holiday food and drink; and share it with those who don't have anything: This day is holy to God. Don't feel bad. The joy of GOD is your strength!"

Selah (pause and reflect)

To some, this scripture may seem an odd one to include in our 100-day "power walk" with God, but I say: "You should look again!" There is a wealth of teaching in just these few lines. For example, one of the most powerful revelations for many will be that the Lord confirms that there <u>are</u> times for us to feast! Praise God! Yes, there are times to enjoy holiday food and drink. (However, this would also indicate that these are special and even sacred times…*not* all the time!)

If you take time to read more in this chapter of Nehemiah, you will see the purpose of the feast: the people had just been brought out of captivity! So, they gathered to hear the Word of the Lord and praise Him! The priests instructed the people to celebrate and glorify God. We are not to feel bad or condemned, but rather to be joyful. When done at the proper time and unto the Lord, feasting will bring both joy and, listen to this…strength!

I actually found these wonderful verses while doing some study of the Word regarding feasting and fasting. I found a common theme woven throughout the scriptures. Both feasting and fasting are meant to bring us into right perspective about God, about food, and about our own selfishness and self-centeredness. For example, our scripture today from Nehemiah tells us to 1) celebrate the day as holy to the Lord, 2) prepare and consume holiday food with joy and 3) share that feast with others – it is not just for you!

Beloved, God made food for your fuel and for your pleasure! He just wants you to be sure you keep them both in balance. Food and drink are not your gods. Neither consuming them nor refraining from them (having too much or too little) should steal your joy!

THE PICTURE OF HEALTH® DAILY POWER PLAN™
Day 30

Proverbs 29:1 (NIV)

> A man who remains stiff-necked after many rebukes will suddenly be destroyed-without remedy.

Proverbs 29:1 (Young's Literal Translation)

> A man often reproved, hardening the neck, is suddenly broken, and there is no healing.

Proverbs 29:1 (The Message)

> For people who hate discipline and only get more stubborn, there'll come a day when life tumbles in and they break, but by then it'll be too late to help them.

Selah (pause and reflect):

Years ago, I was given a ceramic mug with the caption on it, "Your Health...Your Choice". I have kept that all these years as a reminder of how far the Lord has brought me in my life and in my health. I thank the Lord for His mercy and grace that brought me out of the lifestyle that was leading to disease and destruction. He has been faithful to teach me and guide me every step into health and joy like I never dreamed existed! And now, even greater, I have the exceeding joy of seeing that overflow into my children and grandchildren. I see their lives beginning to blossom in health and faith and prosperity in an ever-increasing measure, giving birth to a future the likes of which we never dreamed of or have ever seen. Each day brings such new excitement; I thank God for choosing us to live in this special time.

I have come to understand through the Word of God that He is always lovingly calling us to receive the great gift He has provided for our benefit, now and in the life to come. I can look back and see the places where my life began to change. Three memories in particular stand out. The first was a moment of amazing forgiveness and surrender in December 1994 that opened my heart to let the Lord work in me His purpose. The second was the week in 1997 that a Sunday School class of 5th and 6th graders and I adopted James 1:22 as our motto. (We hung "Just Do It" posters all over the room and never imagined how it would change our lives forever!)

That scripture tells us not to be hearers only, and thereby deceiving ourselves, but to be ***doers*** of the Word. In James 1:25 (NIV) it is written: "But the man who looks intently into the perfect law that gives freedom, and *continues to do this, not forgetting what he has heard, but doing it–he will be blessed in what he does.*" (Emphasis mine.)

Deuteronomy 30:19 tells us that the Lord has set before us life and death, blessings and curses...*choose* life that you and your children shall live. *Choosing is an action*. It is not always easy. But I have found that it was, and is, by choosing, *by doing the Word,* that my life and the lives of many around me have been impacted by the love and power of God in real, tangible, life changing ways. These changes have been in the inner man, but they have been in the outer man as well. Not one area of my life has failed to be redeemed.

What does all this have to do with the Power Verse this week? Just this: The Word of God has given us the choice, the choice I faced in 1994 and perhaps the one you face today. We can continue to repeatedly ignore the correction, discipline, and reproof (given so that you may possess His best for you!) and suddenly one day be destroyed, broken to far to heal. *Or*, we can look into the perfect law that gives freedom, and continue to do it, being blessed in all that we do.

I have lived both ways...blessed is not only better, it is beyond compare, beyond all that I could have asked, thought, or imagined! I pray today that this small bit of testimony will speak to your heart with the Love and the health that awaits your choice.

Oh yes, and that the third distinct moment of change? It was 1999 in a little village in Mexico, miles and light-years away from my former life, when a small class of preschool students and I learned, "Porque fiel es el que prometió*." In English, that means:

(Fear not,) <u>He who promised is faithful</u>. (Hebrews 10:23)

THE PICTURE OF HEALTH®
DAILY POWER PLAN™
Day 31

Galatians 6:7-9 (NLT)

> Don't be misled. Remember that you can't ignore God and get away with it. You will always reap what you sow! Those who live only to satisfy their own sinful desires will harvest the consequences of decay and death. But those who live to please the Spirit will harvest everlasting life from the Spirit. So don't get tired of doing what is good. Don't get discouraged and give up, for we will reap a harvest of blessing at the appropriate time.

Selah (pause and reflect)

Have you checked your crops lately? What have you been sowing? If it was weeds (destruction, self-indulgence)... well, get busy and yank them up and plant something new! And if you have been sowing good seeds for good health, water them and get ready to harvest!

Right here in front of us we have the promise. But you can't give up! You can't get tired of doing what is good! And...you can't continue to ignore the truth that God is trying to bring you about your health! For those who do ignore Him, the King James Version of this scripture says God is not mocked! They will reap the consequences of decay and death.

Oh! But beloved, not us! We will listen and live to please God. We <u>will reap</u> the harvest of life!

The Picture of Health®
Daily Power Plan™
Day 32

Jeremiah 29:11 (KJV)

> For I know the thoughts that I think toward you, saith the LORD, thoughts of peace, and not of evil, to give you an expected end.

Selah (pause and reflect)

An expected end. Think about it: God has always had an expected end in mind for my life and yours...***an outcome of His choosing.***

Now, you may have already known that or you may not have. But have you ever stopped to realize that, because His Word never returns to Him void or without accomplishing that for which it was sent, the outcome He first expected for me (and for you) **shall** come to pass!

What is that outcome? It is the fulfillment of His purpose for me, the reason I was created! 1st Corinthians 6:19-20, tells us that we are not our own, but we were bought with a price, *for His purpose*. That purpose is my "expected end".

Of course, with God we always have a choice. It is through our choices of willingness and obedience to receive from Him that the power of heaven moves to cause His Word to be fulfilled in our lives (Is 1:19). First, we must accept His gift, that payment for our salvation, healing, and deliverance. Second, we must be doers of the Word. As we do these things, we permit and invite God to work that expected end in our lives.

Why waste another day? Let's get in faith about this and start living by His thoughts; the thoughts the Word says are *to prosper us and to give us a hope and a future!* Let's start living out our "expected end"! And, as my pastor likes to ask, "How will you know if you are really in faith about it?" You get excited about it coming to pass!

I am greatly excited to be walking in *the outcome of His choosing* for my life!

How about you?

THE PICTURE OF HEALTH® DAILY POWER PLAN™

Day 33

Zechariah 6:12-15 (AMP)

> And say to him, Thus says the Lord of hosts: [You, Joshua] behold (look at, keep in sight, watch) the Man [the Messiah] whose name is the Branch, for He shall grow up in His place and He shall build the [true] temple of the Lord.
>
> Yes, [you are building a temple of the Lord, but] it is He Who shall build the [true] temple of the Lord, and He shall bear the honor and glory [as of the only begotten of the Father] and shall sit and rule upon His throne. And He shall be a Priest upon His throne, and the counsel of peace shall be between the two [offices—Priest and King]. And the [other] crown shall be [credited] to Helem (Heldai), to Tobijah, and to Jedaiah, and to the kindness and favor of Josiah the son of Zephaniah, and shall be in the temple of the Lord for a reminder and memorial.
>
> And those who are far off shall come and help build the temple of the Lord, and you shall know (recognize and understand) that the Lord sent me [Zechariah] to you. And [your part in this] shall come to pass if you will diligently obey the voice of the Lord your God.

Selah (pause and reflect)

Yesterday, I seemed to be surrounded by too many selfish people who were pulling on me, whining about first one thing and then another, and oblivious to anyone but themselves. These are the same self-absorbed people who are still making excuses as to why they had not yet done the last thing the Lord prompted them to do. You know, "suckers", people who try to suck all the anointing and life out of you because they are too lazy to activate faith for themselves.

Ever have a day like that? Well, to be honest, it was flat getting on my nerves! Just about that time, I read a note in a class member's chart. The person writing had already made a substantial recovery of health, but had a few private questions for me. In answering them, I noticed these comments: "My only New Year's resolution is to get closer to the Lord - trust Him more. That is the reason my (health is improving) - HIM."

Oh how that deeply touched me. Just when I needed it, this lovely heart truly encouraged me in the Lord. I thanked my God and said, "(This person) gets it, Lord. Somebody really does get it". I thought to myself, "Yes and this person is reaping the real, lasting results as evidence." It is the difference between *knowing in your head*, intellectually or perhaps religiously, that He is the source and truly having *revelation in your heart by faith* that **He is the source**. One is blind. One can see.

As we attempt to walk in health, sometimes we get caught up in "doing" and start thinking that we did this on our own. You know, like we "got healthy" by our works. Once the results start showing, it is often easy to forget that it is He who deserves the glory…and the thanks. Yes, we surrender and obey the Word, but it is the Lord who builds the temple, not us.

If you were to take a minute or two to look at King Nebuchadnezzar in Daniel Chapter 4, in verse 2, you would find him telling of the Lord's greatness, the things *the Lord* had done toward him. However, by verse 29, just 12 months later, we see the same King boasting about what *he* (the King) had done. The Word says at that moment, as pride stepped in, the kingdom departed from him and he became as an animal. Yuck!

That is what happens to people who fail to recognize who it is that redeems their health. They become forgetful of the miracle that saved them. Oftentimes they lose all the progress they made in their health and develop even worse diseases or problems than they had before. It is written that "pride goeth before destruction" (Proverbs 16:18 KJV). The moment we take the task on ourselves, the burden becomes heavy and the goal unreachable; any success is swallowed up in our pride.

So, beloved, remember who it is that has redeemed you. And just as He sent those words of encouragement to me, He has promised in The Word that He will send people to help you. Your part in this shall come to pass if you will diligently obey the voice of the Lord your God. **When you acknowledge God as the source and give Him all the glory, the results will come and the results will last.**

THE PICTURE OF HEALTH® DAILY POWER PLAN™

Day 34

Jeremiah 31:12 (NLT)

> They will come home and sing songs of joy on the heights of Jerusalem. They will be radiant because of the many gifts the LORD has given them—the good crops of wheat, wine, and oil, and the healthy flocks and herds. Their life will be like a watered garden, and all their sorrows will be gone.

Selah (pause and reflect)

"Hi! How are you?" How many times will someone ask you that today? Most of us will be asked that question at least 5 times each day, possibly 20 or more depending on where you go that day and how many people you greet! What is your usual response? "Fine." Or, "Good."

Did you realize that every time someone asks you that question you have the opportunity to give a testimony of the Lord's goodness? I bet you never even thought about it. If the truth were known, most people don't even stop long enough to hear your answer. Or even funnier is the person who answers you with "Good!" before you even ask how they are! That is because people are basically self-absorbed. Another common reason they don't wait for an answer is because they are afraid you might start in on a sob-story!

I'd like to challenge you today to begin replying with words that strengthen you and the hearer. Sure you might get a few shocked looks, but everyone needs a little more fun in their lives! The next time someone asks, "How are you?" Tell him or her, "I am bursting with life!" (See? Doesn't that put a smile on your face just to say it?) Or you could respond, "Radiant! I am well-watered by the hand of God!"

You may be laughing now, but laughter is good medicine! Try it! And watch the doors open for you to tell others what He has done in your life and in your body!

THE PICTURE OF HEALTH® DAILY POWER PLAN™
Day 35

Luke 4:4 (King James Version)

> And Jesus answered him, saying, It is written, That man shall not live by bread alone, but by every word of God.

Selah (pause and reflect)

In the days, hours, and moments just before the greatest event of His life, Christ encountered the greatest temptations of His life. He was physically hungry, emotionally tired, and separated from all those around him. He knew that the days ahead would hold the announcement of his true purpose and ultimately his expected end. Jesus was tempted to give in. But He did *not* give in.

This is particularly important for many of you to hear today. Right now, this day, there are those of you who are standing on the threshold of your purpose in God. As the fullness of that purpose approaches, *we*, like Jesus, must refuse to give in to the flesh and the carnal desires of our physical body. We must *not* seek to satisfy ourselves or indulge in natural cravings, but rather, as God leads, we must fast (do without something) in order to press in closer to Him and feast on the Word of God.

Does that mean we should all fast from all food as He did for 40 days? <u>Absolutely not.</u> Only very few people in the Bible were ever called upon by God to do that. However, the Lord may lead you to fast from a certain food or foods that master you or control you. It may be like Daniel for

10 days to strengthen you or 21 days to bring you revelation. It may be like Esther, for three days to break down strongholds in your life. It could be just one meal spent in the Word rather than the kitchen.

The point of fasting is not the absence of food but the presence of the Word.

The Word can break you free from self-indulgence and disobedience. The Word can sharpen your awareness of His presence and His power to sustain you. The Word can prepare you for the next move of His Spirit in your life.

> And Jesus answered him, saying, "It is written that man shall not live by bread alone, but by every word of God."

THE PICTURE OF HEALTH®
DAILY POWER PLAN™
Day 36

Galatians 5:1 (NLT)

> So Christ has really set us free. Now make sure that you stay free, and don't get tied up again in slavery to the law.

Selah (pause and reflect)

The Word in John 8:32 (NLT) says, "You will know the truth, and the truth will make you free". And Christ said, "I am the Way, the Truth, and the Life." Because Christ *is* the Truth, He is **the answer** to all bondage and slavery, to all torment and torture (including all sickness and disease).

Beloved, you and I, and others around us on this journey, are finding this Truth daily in the Word of God, and it is making us free! Free now and forever more from diets, death, destruction, and disease!

Our lives should be extraordinarily joyful because of this freedom, but I sense in my spirit that some of you today can't feel that freedom. Some of you want to be joyful, but the current fact is that you are burdened and discouraged.

If that is you, if you are not feeling free, the answer is to feed yourself on more of the truth. If you struggle with your self-image or your ability to remain faithful and steadfast, then those are signs that you are feeling the effects of deception in your life. Deception is a device of the enemy to kill, steal, and destroy you. Deception is designed to bring bondage. The way out, the way to possess freedom now and forever is living in and by His TRUTH, which is the Word of God.

How exactly does one do that? It isn't by trying to be good. It isn't by doing religious things or works. There is only one way. Romans 12:2 (NLT) says,

> Don't copy the behavior and customs of this world, but let God transform you into a new person by changing the way you think. Then you will know what God wants you to do, and you will know how good and pleasing and perfect his will really is.

How does He change the way you think? By renewing the mind through the washing of the water of the Word. You bathe your heart and mind in the Word of God. You look up scripture in the Word that tells you who you are in Christ and commit those to heart and to memory. You <u>don't</u> copy the behavior or customs of this world!

For example, you are a child of the Most High God, a joint-heir with Christ, a King's kid, royalty. Your prayers are a sweet smelling savor to Him. You are more than a conqueror in Christ and can do all things through Him, which strengthens you. You are the one He adores. You are God's favored child. You are the redeemed of the Lord; you have been rescued, bought with a price, restored, and recreated in Him. You are a cherished, holy priesthood unto Him. He causes all things to work together for your good because you love Him and you are called according to His purpose.

I could keep going, but you need to do some of this for yourselves. You can start by finding the verses that the above truths come from. Train yourself to get into His love letters to you and ***find yourself in His Word***. Did you know that John the Baptist found himself in the Word (Mark 1, Luke 1, and Matthew 3) as "the one calling in the wilderness" preparing the way for the Lord? Do you recall that in Luke 4:16-21, Jesus even found himself in the Word and revealed himself to others through reading the passage from what is now Isaiah 61:1-2?

The second half of the scripture for today tells <u>us</u> to see to it that *we* stay free. We do that by knowing who He is and who we are in Him. We do that by being doers of the Word. We don't copy the customs of this world. We find ourselves in the Word!

For extra help in this, I am going to give you an assignment that one of my Bible School teachers gave me. I want you to take time this week to write a paper. Make it one or two pages long, containing statements from the Word telling you who you are. Put a copy where you will see it daily and speak it to yourself. As these truths become written on the tablets of your heart, you will see great joy, confidence, and yes, health, blossom in your life, Spirit, Soul, and Body!

You are the Body of Christ, the church triumphant, adorned in splendor, walking in the unforced rhythms of grace, destined to rule and reign in this life and the life to come!

THE PICTURE OF HEALTH®
DAILY POWER PLAN™
Day 37

Luke 8:18 (NIV)

> Therefore consider carefully how you listen. Whoever has will be given more; whoever does not have, even what he thinks he has will be taken from him.

Selah (pause and reflect)

LISTEN. That seems easy enough. Most of us would say, "I *am* listening." Before you decide that, take another look at the verse. The verse says:

*"Consider carefully **how you listen**."*

Here is a test that might help: Examine the results of your listening. Does the evidence that presents itself indicate you are partaking in the victory He provided? Do you have peace, health, joy, and abundance? Or are there areas that don't show so much victory? Perhaps you have not been careful about how you listen in those areas.

Here's what I mean. Let's just use the classes I teach for an example. Many come and the Word of God changes their lives forever. They reclaim their health and discover freedom and joy like never before. But there are others, fewer, but still there are some, who come (sometimes over and over) and walk out without it ever changing their lives. I can see those people months or years later and still no evidence of change, no health, no increase in joy, and no increase in freedom. More often than not, their health is even worse than before.

What is the difference?

I wanted to know. I knew the Word tells us in Hosea 4:6 that His people perish from lack of knowledge. But I could not explain why, after the Lord brought people life-changing, life-saving knowledge, there seemed to be no change. I went back to the Word and found something I had never seen before.

This is what Hosea 4:6 (NIV) <u>really</u> says: (emphasis added is mine)

...my people are destroyed from lack of knowledge.

Because you have rejected knowledge,

I also reject you as my priests;

Because you have ignored the law of your God,

I also will ignore your children.

What an answer. The ones who perish have ***rejected the knowledge*** the Lord tried to bring to them! As a result, they *and their children* were rejected.

It is the ones who come **teachable**, who want to learn, and who *do what the Lord gives them revelation on,* these are the ones who are increased and who prosper in their spirit, soul, and body. Step by step they walk in the light (revelation, knowledge) they are being given. And, because they make a sincere effort to hear Him and obey Him, they are given even more light, more revelation about their health.

You are that one. How do I know that? Because you are here every day checking the Power Plan, aren't you? Listen to me. You are being faithful to walk in the light He is giving you and He will increase you because of it. You don't have to be perfect. Continue to consider carefully how you listen. Be humble, be teachable, be faithful, and *He will increase both you and your children.*

THE PICTURE OF HEALTH®
DAILY POWER PLAN™
Day 38

Psalm 19:7-8 (The Message)

> The revelation of GOD is whole
>
> and pulls our lives together.
>
> The signposts of GOD are clear
>
> and point out the right road.
>
> The life-maps of GOD are right,
>
> showing the way to joy.
>
> The directions of GOD are plain
>
> and easy on the eyes.

Selah (pause and reflect)

Oh! Give thanks to the Lord whose mercy endures forever! This wonderful Psalm is exactly what I wanted to say to you today! I wanted to testify of His goodness. As I prayed about what to say, He blessed me by leading me to this beautiful description in the Psalms.

I tell you the truth it is He who pulls my life together. It is He who points out the right road and gives me a map showing me the way to joy. It is He who makes it plain so that even I can understand and it is not difficult to see. The light in my eyes, the love in my life, the purpose of my days...it is He who has placed them there.

Have you felt the desire stirring in you for these things of the Lord? He will do it! I will tell you right now, people come too late to convince me that He won't. I am a wholly new creation in every aspect of my life and wouldn't go back for anything in this entire world! I am sold out and never drawing back again. I am telling you, He is faithful and the Word is true. This passage is reality for me every day. It can and will be fulfilled in your life too as you yield to Him and act upon the Word of God!

You can make this passage personal today. You do that by saying the words to yourself out loud, putting yourself ("me", "to me", and "my") in the passage so that it becomes your confession. But listen, it is more than just a positive confession. You must make it the words of your heart. As you do, the power of the Word of God will work in you to bring it to pass, activated by your faith in Him. When it does, give Him the glory and testify of His goodness to others!

The Picture of Health®
Daily Power Plan™
Day 39

Isaiah 48:17-19 (New International Version)

> This is what the LORD says- your Redeemer, the Holy One of Israel: "I am the LORD your God, who teaches you what is best for you, who directs you in the way you should go. If only you had paid attention to my commands, your peace would have been like a river, your righteousness like the waves of the sea. Your descendants would have been like the sand, your children like its numberless grains; their name would never be cut off nor destroyed from before me."

Selah (pause and reflect)

Have you noticed that our studies keep coming back to a certain recurring message from the Lord? I see that He keeps leading us back to scripture after scripture that show us how to flourish, be in health, have victory, and live in blessing. You know, I have reached a time in my life where that is what I want more than anything else in life! Well, except perhaps for my children and grandchildren to have it in even greater measure! And with great wonder and awe, I am watching that happen in my life.

I mean, just look at this: The Lord is personally telling me (each of us) that **He will teach me what is best for m**e. How easy does that make it?! And it is true. For example, just how do you think I have learned all that I teach you in The Picture of Health™? *He taught it to me.* Sometimes, often, He just drops it in my brain! It is the coolest thing! It is really funny when there is a super-educated person in class, you know, an "intellectual". It just drives the scholars crazy trying to figure out how I know these things! They just don't get it: *I don't know these things*...but *He does*!

How do I do what I do? **The Lord directs me in the way I should go**, so I don't have to wander or be confused. He tells me that **because I pay attention to His commands, my peace is like a river and my righteousness like the waves of the sea!** That means to me that I have ever flowing, life-giving oxygen coming in to my life every day from the Spirit of God causing my spirit, soul, and body to be strong and healthy.

This passage also confirms to me the greatest of all my desires: if I pay attention to put into practice all His commands, my children and all my descendants will be uncountable and theirs names will always be before the Lord! That is worthy of a shout and a dance too!

I can't imagine that it gets any better than that! But you know what? It actually does get better than that! He enlarges my tent and makes me a blessing indeed as He gives the opportunity to share His goodness with you.

If you need knowledge, direction, peace, salvation for you and/or your family members, or anything else, it is all in there. All you have to do is believe, receive, confess it with your mouth, and live to walk it out. My life is a living testimony of His truth and faithfulness...yours can be too. His Word accomplishes that for which it was sent. His love never fails. I invite you to take it as your Word from Him today.

THE PICTURE OF HEALTH®
DAILY POWER PLAN™
Day 40

1 Chronicles 29:3 (KJV)

> Moreover, because I have set my affection to the house of my God, I have of mine own proper good, of gold and silver, which I have given to the house of my God, over and above all that I have prepared for the holy house.

Selah (pause and reflect)

Remember how I have been encouraging you to find yourself in the Word? As I was reading 1 Chronicles one day, the Lord gave me a very clear glimpse of my purpose. It has helped me so much in my health walk that I want to share it with you. I believe it will help you as you seek to find yourself in His Word.

If you read the whole account surrounding this passage in 1 Chronicles, the scene refers to the building of the temple. Interestingly enough, we see that David was given the plan (or "the pattern") for the new temple building, a building of lavish beauty to glorify God. David amassed great wealth and laid it up for the building of this awesome structure. But he was *not* allowed to build it. <u>*David was a pattern-giver.*</u> David asked, "Who will?" David presented the pattern to the people and rallied them to step up and be a part of a most extraordinary opportunity.

The record of this whole process is undeniably a type and shadow of our care of the temple, which is now our physical body. This is where I found myself. Our primary commission is to carry the good news of the Kingdom of God to the entire world. To be more specific, much like David our mission through *The Picture of Health®* is to present to you *the pattern*.

David wasn't only giving the people of God a pep-talk so they would feel warm and fuzzy. (And neither am I.) He was calling them to action. He was rallying them to show their affection with action. And so am I. The first step in rebuilding the glorious temple of God begins in your heart. This was the call David issued to the people and I issue it to you today:

Have you set your affection on the house (dwelling place) of your God?

THE PICTURE OF HEALTH®
DAILY POWER PLAN™
Day 41

1 Chronicles 29:5 (KJV)

>...for the gold work and the silver work, and for all the work to be done by the craftsmen. Now, who is willing to consecrate himself today to the LORD?

<u>Selah (pause and reflect)</u>

In our study yesterday we found that it was God who prepared the pattern (the blueprint) for the glorious temple. It was God who supplied David with the resources and laid it upon David's heart to issue the call. But who was it that responded?

Solomon responded to that call. *Solomon was the "temple builder".* He <u>received</u> the pattern and made it a reality. He and the people consecrated themselves unto God and stepped up to the mark of the high calling. Down to every detail, no expense was spared, no shortcuts taken. The temple was built in "glorious splendor"!

In response to Solomon's expression of affection, the Lord blessed Solomon in wisdom and riches. The splendor of his house and the measure of his wisdom was so renowned that the Queen of Sheba came from across the earth to see him. Was it about Solomon? No. Even this woman of the world recognized that the prosperity and excellence of Solomon's life were a testimony to the goodness and power of God. The Bible records this response from her in 2 Chronicles 9:8: "Praise be to the Lord your God, who has delighted in you".

You are to be a living memorial unto His Majesty!

Solomon's temple and the wisdom by which he ruled ignited the interest of the world around him. We are also to be witnesses of the Kingdom of God at work and alive in us! 2 Corinthians 5:20 says we are ambassadors for Christ. The reality and the goodness of God at work in our lives should be proof of whose message we carry.

People should look at you and know that God is good!

The Amplified Bible asks it this way: "Who will offer willingly to fill his hand and consecrate it today to the Lord like one consecrating himself to the priesthood?"

Is it the desire of your heart to give over and above what you have ever offered Him before? Are you willing to take that step and be accountable unto Him? Are you ready to be a "temple builder"? Now is time when the opportunity is being presented. Step up and prepare the holy house of God!

THE PICTURE OF HEALTH®
DAILY POWER PLAN™
Day 42

1 Thessalonians 5:23 (AMP)

> And may the God of peace Himself sanctify you through and through [separate you from profane things, make you pure and wholly consecrated to God]; and may your spirit and soul and body be preserved sound and complete [and found] blameless at the coming of our Lord Jesus Christ (the Messiah).

Selah (pause and reflect)

Beloved, we have walked together for six weeks now. I sense today you need some encouragement and to renew your strength. I exhort you to not give up! Don't quit! Always be mindful that this is a journey to divine health, a journey that leads us into the very heart of God.

Please know that as we have been sharing together the Word in our daily intimate time with Him, and with each other, I have been praying that each of us, me included, will be drawn into that place of blessing, to understand what is our glorious inheritance through Jesus Christ, which He purchased, as a gift, for all who will believe on Him and be saved.

As I tell all new participants in *The Picture of Health*® wellness and nutrition classes, when you made the decision to sign up and show up, or in this case, to open up (to this page), you must have been seeking relief from something. Why give up when the relief is at hand?

Some of you seek relief from sickness and disease. For others, the something is your weight - too much or too little - perhaps an eating disorder of some kind. For others, your "something" is depression, mood swings, menopause, anger, or stress. For still others, it is a lack of knowledge. (We'll look at *that one* again later!) Many of you have already begun to sense the conviction of heart to know (and do) God's Word in greater measure, specifically in regard to your body, the temple of the Holy Spirit.

*Regardless of what it is you seek relief from, God's Word **will** reveal the answer.*

How can I be so sure? Because no matter what you, the world, or any doctor, have named the problem...The Name of the solution remains the same! His Name - the Name of Jesus Christ - is the Name above all names, and, therefore, the Name above *all* sickness and disease.

By faith and obedience to the Word of God, you can be made whole, *completely healed*, just like the man described in Acts 3:16, where it was said of him, "By faith in the name of Jesus, this man whom you see and know was made strong. It is Jesus' name and the faith that comes through him that has given this complete healing to him, as you can all see."

I ask you to spend some time today, alone with the Lord, rededicating your heart to our studies. Remember that every day you should be walking in your covenant with Him through the Blood of Christ and the Holy Spirit that dwells in you.

It is written in Psalms 119:133, Proverbs 4:11, and Proverbs 3:6:

He orders your footsteps; He directs your paths.

It is no coincidence, and it is no accident, that you have found, or been given, this book at this time. Beloved, He desires above all else that you prosper and be in health, even as your soul prospers. You should rejoice! For this is the day of your salvation! This is the day for your healing! This, child of The Most High God is your day of deliverance! This is the day *you live* a life of victory - fullness in Him - spirit, soul, and body!

I'll be praying with you and for you from the Word: (Ephesians 1:17-19 NIV)

Glorious Father, God of our Lord Jesus Christ, I pray for each of these, your children, that you will give them *the Spirit of wisdom and revelation,* **so that** they may *know You better.* I pray also that *the eyes of their hearts may be enlightened* in order *that they may know the hope to which You have called them, the riches of Your glorious inheritance* in the saints, and *Your incomparably great power for us who believe.*

According to that which you, Lord, have spoken, let it be so. In Jesus' Name, Amen

THE PICTURE OF HEALTH®
DAILY POWER PLAN™
Day 43

Hebrews 7:18-19, 28 (New International Version)

> The former regulation is set aside because it was weak and useless (for the law made nothing perfect), and a better hope is introduced, by which we draw near to God.
>
> For the law appoints as high priests men who are weak; but the oath, which came after the law, appointed the Son, who has been made perfect forever.

Selah (pause and reflect)

Here it is straight so that there is no misunderstanding: the law made nothing perfect. Because it was based on regulations and control, it was weak and useless. That is a great description of a diet! Whether it is a diet to lose weight, a diet to lower your cholesterol, a heart diet, a diabetes diet, a what-ever-you-call-it diet, they are, by design, based on regulations.

**ized*Diets are not healthy, but are designed instead to keep you in bondage.*

Our scripture tells us that the law appoints priests who are weak, *subject to law to maintain order*. This is the same principle that modern diets use in their attempt to "maintain order" in your body. And they fail for the same reasons: they are weak and useless because they don't get to the heart of the issue. Incidentally, this truth even applies to the dietary <u>regulations</u> of the Old Testament if looked at or performed *alone* without grace. We'll look at that again another day, but today let's suffice it to point out that these regulations have been set aside.

We no longer have to chase first one diet, program, or fad after another trying to find something that will work. We have a strong, perfected Priest who operates with the law fulfilled *inside* through grace. He is the one who through God's great love has been made perfect forever! And as we let Him, He will perfect His love in us as well.

Beloved, "God has chosen to make known...the glorious riches of this mystery, which is Christ in you, the hope of glory." (Colossians 1:27 NIV) That is good news, beloved! Get a hold of it! The next time the diet mentality encroaches on your thoughts, remind yourself that we *draw near to God* through Christ, <u>not based on regulation</u> but on the ***power of an indestructible life!***

> His divine power has given us everything we need for life and godliness through our knowledge of him who called us by his own glory and goodness. (2 Peter 1:3 NIV)

The Picture of Health® Daily Power Plan™

Day 44

Romans 8:11 (NIV)

> And if the Spirit of him who raised Jesus from the dead is living in you, he who raised Christ from the dead will also give life to your mortal bodies through his Spirit, who lives in you.

Selah (pause and reflect)

We learned in yesterday's walk that we *draw near to God* through Christ, not based on regulation but on the ***power of an indestructible life!*** I believe this is one of the most often missed parts of His love among the body of Christ. Think about it! In us abides the power of an indestructible life. The same power that raised Christ from the dead lives in you! Wow! Now *that* is power!

But are you applying that power? Today we see in scripture that it is through that power working in us by which *He quickens our mortal body*. People tend to accept the provision of eternal life, yet fail to lay hold of the truth whereby that same power can have breathe life into our bodies *now*.

Because of His great love for us, He laid down His life for us. He set His love on us and provided the way of salvation, healing, and deliverance (Luke 4:18-21). This is available in this life *and* the life to come for every person who would believe and confess Him as Lord and Savior. He does it *with purpose*. The Bible declares in 1 John 3:16 *why*. He desires that we live in health in this life as well as for eternity so that, as He did for us, we can do for others, laying down our lives for our brothers.

Don't unhook from me now. I know that many people shut right down at the thought of this health walk being about someone other than you. If that is you and you are saying, "Yea, yea, but this is about weight for me. I do plenty for Christ at church. I am not neglecting my call. This part is just a personal thing. I need to diet or to workout and I will be fine." Or, "I have to get rid of this disease before I can do anything for someone else." Or even perhaps, "I love God. But I am doing this right now so I look good for my wedding."

Will you receive the correction of the Lord in love? These two areas of your life, your relationship with the Lord and the state of your physical body, are not separate and they are not two different areas. You are participating in a lie from the devil as long as you hold to that belief. How's that? Because the enemy knows that view of one's body will keep you from experiencing the fullness of God's blessing! You are meant to be blessed spirit, soul, and body in this life and the life to come. Any measure of that blessing the devil can steal from you through deception or your own rebellion, believe me, he will.

But I am going to believe that is not you! I believe you want the fullness God has purchased for you and that you are mature enough by now to hear this. So stick with me and we will all come up in the power that is in us. Be willing to let go of your past feelings and *learn His way to victory*.

There is a great commission given for every child of God. Your mission is to actively **display** the love and goodness of God in every area of your life (including and most especially your body) so that others are drawn to Him. The Bible declares that *it is the love of God that turns men to repentance.*

Our very lives, even our bodies, are to be proof of His love and goodness.

Remember what we studied about Solomon? I haven't gotten off the subject of health and life in your physical body. In fact, that is exactly what I am addressing. If the Lord raised Christ from the dead, and He did, He can and will quicken your physical body to be the size, shape, and weight that glorifies Him. He is only waiting on you to yield and invite Him to be Lord of your body too.

Beloved, everyone who sees you doesn't get the opportunity to know your heart. More often than not, people who pass by you only have the opportunity to judge God's work in your life by the outward man. It isn't the most important part, but it is a walking billboard! It is a reflection of the man inside. *If you don't possess health and life in your mortal body, you will be much less able to be a witness of His love to others.*

If you are sick, diseased, depressed and anxious all the time, or burdened by weight problems and eating disorders, your body does *not* testify that He heals. If we are the "poster child" for obesity or anorexia, the result of our rebellion reflects on how others perceive God.

Beloved, if you are born-again in Christ, the Holy Spirit is alive in you to cause your body to be more glorious than Solomon's temple. The power to quicken your mortal body is within you right now. It only takes one moment to surrender every area of your life and reap the harvest of health that is yours in the Kingdom of God. If you don't have that, you can receive it now. If you are ready for a quickening in your body, pray this with me:

> *Thank you Lord for saving, healing, and delivering me out of the darkness into your great Light. Come Lord Jesus, I surrender my whole life to you. I repent of my rebellion and yield my will to yours. Renew my mind in your Word. Quicken my mortal body and fulfill in me that for which I was created. Amen.*

That settles it. Know that His power is changing your body even as you finish our "walk" with Him today. Don't ever pick up the reigns again yourself. Be led now by His direction and the desire that your body glorify Him. You are now an ambassador for Him. Lay hold of the gift of Christ by the power of the Holy Spirit. Let His power be manifest in you for all to see, bringing glory to God, for that is why you are quickened!

THE PICTURE OF HEALTH®
DAILY POWER PLAN™
Day 45

Proverbs 4: 4-7 (NKJV)

He also taught me, and said to me:

"Let your heart retain my words; Keep my commands, and live.

Get wisdom! Get understanding!

Do not forget, nor turn away from the words of my mouth.

Do not forsake her, and she will preserve you;

Love her, and she will keep you.

Wisdom is the principal thing; Therefore get wisdom.

And in all your getting, get understanding."

Selah (pause and reflect)

This passage is like a mini-lesson at the feet of God. He instructs us today (through the scriptures) exactly what it is that will produce health and life in our bodies: His Word.

As you meditate on God's Word, take heed to His instruction:

1) *Retain His Word* in your heart - not just your ears or your head, but in your heart.

2) *Keep His commands* - be doer's of the Word that He gives you.

3) *Get wisdom and understanding* - don't just read the verse and go on...endeavor to understand what it is that God wants to speak *to you* on *that day.* "Get" is an action verb!

4) *Do not forget nor turn away.* Wisdom, the skillful use of knowledge, will *preserve* you and *keep* you!

The Lord is teaching us how to do this day by day. He, Almighty God, is leading us on the path to fullness. Apply what you are learning. "*Get it!*"

THE PICTURE OF HEALTH®
DAILY POWER PLAN™

Day 46

Proverbs 4:13-15 (KJV)

Take fast hold of instruction; let her not go: keep her; for she is thy life.

Enter not into the path of the wicked, and go not in the way of evil men.

Avoid it, pass not by it, turn from it, and pass away.

Selah (pause and reflect)

I learned something from Dr. Jim Perkins, a dear pastor of mine from years ago, which has helped me greatly ever since. Actually, he and his family taught me many things about the Lord and the love of God that impacted my life forever, but this one thing I'll share with you today: "**Decide in advance**."

He told me just shortly after I truly came to know Christ in a personal relationship that if I settled the decision in advance that Sunday was set aside to worship the Lord - in church with the fellowship of other believers - then when Sunday came, it would have no bearing on me if it were raining, snowing, if I was sleepy, on vacation, etc. My decision would already have been made.

I believe this same wisdom has come to my remembrance and helped me in my health walk as well. See, I decide or "settle it" in advance what I am going to eat at a certain restaurant. I decide in advance that I am not stopping for donuts, even when the sign does say "hot"! I settle the decision in advance as to what I will snack on or drink when I travel and I prepare for it. And, along the same lines, if I suspect I will be seeing someone who may not be the easiest to be around or who may not be friendly, I verbally, out loud, instruct myself and decide in advance that I will walk in love no matter what occurs.

Our scripture for today tells us that the instruction of the Lord is *life*. If we are to consistently walk in that life, we must consciously, decisively turn away from our old path. We must hold fast to the Lord's path and instruction for our lives; we must avoid old destructive ways and not even go near them.

So, settle it. Decide in advance. Then, let His grace give you the strength to follow through with your decision.

The Picture of Health® Daily Power Plan™

Day 47

Proverbs 4:10 (KJV)

> Hear, O my son, and receive my sayings;
> and the years of thy life shall be many.

Selah (pause and reflect)

Did you know that it is God's will for you and me to live a long, satisfying life? It is. Look with me in the Word and I will prove it to you. First, we must know that the Word of God says (at least six times in the KJV) that every matter shall be established by the testimony of two or three witnesses. So, I didn't just find one verse about long life and pull it out of context. No, there are over nineteen (19) witnesses[1] in the Word establishing that it is God's desire to give you a good, long life! And, that is if you only use those two words to describe it. I found scripture upon scripture that directly correlate holding fast to His precepts or instructions - keeping His commandments - and having a good, long life!

For example, in addition to our daily scripture above, Proverbs 3:1-2 (KJV) also says, "My son, forget not my law; but let thine heart keep my commandments: For length of days, and long life, and peace, shall they add to thee." God also speaks to us of having a long, satisfying life in Psalm 91:14-16 (KJV):

> Because he hath set his love upon me, therefore will I deliver him: I will set him on high, because he hath known my name. He

shall call upon me, and I will answer him: I will be with him in trouble; I will deliver him, and honour him. With long life will I satisfy him, and shew him my salvation.

If these things are true, should someone ask, "Why then is the average life span in the United States 75.37 years[2]?" That is in sharp contrast to how long people lived before the days of Noah! Granted, some of the changes that took place in the natural earth after the fall of Adam and Eve prevent us from living that long now. But if you study it out, you will see that the primary reason so many die so young is that each promise of a good, *long life is predicated upon one's keeping His commands* (being a doer of the Word). Bless the Lord for teaching us to be doers of the Word! Amen!

Listen how the Lord describes a long life: "length of days", "full age", "fullness of years", and, "as the days of trees." And, we find that Genesis 6:3 tells us that man's days shall be one hundred and twenty years! That is what Dr. Ray and I will be having if the Lord tarries His Second Coming, 120 years!

Now that we are armed with this revelation of God's Truth and we have faithfully purposed to be doers of the Word of God, I challenge you to set your sights on God's best for your lives! Let's agree together with the Word to renew our minds in regard to having not only a long life, but also a *satisfying, full, abundant life, rich in the rewards of God*!

Additional passages for study: Psalm 21:4; Genesis 25:8; Job 5:26; Proverbs 3:2, 16; Proverbs 22:4; Isaiah 65:20-22

[1] NLT - about 19 times, KJV - about 8 times, NIV about 10 times

[2] Sources: U.S. Decennial Life Tables for 1989-1991 Vol. II Sate Life Tables #41.

THE PICTURE OF HEALTH®
DAILY POWER PLAN™
Day 48

John 6:63 (AMP)

> It is the Spirit Who gives life [He is the Life-giver]; the flesh conveys no benefit whatever [there is no profit in it]. The words (truths) that I have been speaking to you are spirit and life.

Selah (pause and reflect)

My heart rejoices and I thank God today for you! Your faithfulness to seek His way in reclaiming your health is an inspiration to me. It is so exciting to me that every day we are, together, growing in His Word and drawing nearer to fully possessing His best and His abundance in our lives!

As you spend time with Him today, let the scriptures reassure you that the Word you have been consuming daily <u>*will not fail*</u> to produce that for which it was sent. Every day that you come here to spend time with Him and in His Word, you not only grow spiritually, but your physical body gets filled with more life, becoming stronger and healthier day by day. Proverbs 4:22 (NIV) tells us that

> ***God's Word is life to those who find it and health to a man's whole body.***

He has given us The Way to health in our whole body. Stand steadfast in your pursuit of Him, holding fast to His instruction, being a doer of His Word, and He will see to it that life and physical health are added unto you.

THE PICTURE OF HEALTH®
DAILY POWER PLAN™
Day 49

Isaiah 55:2 (New International Version)

"Why spend money on what is not bread,

and your labor on what does not satisfy?

Listen, listen to me, and eat what is good,

and your soul will delight in the richest of fare."

Selah (pause and reflect)

Have you been feeling unsatisfied? Are you at unrest with yourself or displeased with your progress, your health, size, shape, or weight? The Lord counsels us in this passage from Isaiah 55:2 to check our focus. Write down your thoughts, what has been going around in your head lately then examine them to see what the main word(s) used is or the recurring theme is.

Is it, for example, "I"? That would mean you are inward focused on yourself rather than the Lord. Is the theme of the thoughts "my weight, this weight, the weight"? Then your focus is on the weight, not on the Lord's ability to show you how to remove it! Perhaps it is on certain symptoms or pain rather than the healing power that is at work inside you? Or are you focused on what you don't like, what doesn't taste good, what isn't easy or tingly to your flesh? The Lord has the answer to all of these gripes!

The real question is...will you receive what He is teaching you and do it?

His answer is sure every time. He tells us: listen. Listen to me. Eat what is good and your soul - your mind, will, and emotions - will delight in the riches of fare!

Check your heart by doing the writing exercise mentioned above. Ask a family member or close friend to tell you what you say and talk most about. (Now, you'll have to receive what they say with thanks and not rebellion. And you'll also have to remember not to attack them when they honestly answer you!) Ask those who love you and see. Do you tell yourself that you are "really trying" when really you are completely resisting His Word? Are you eager to hear him or pretending that is not His voice? Do you really want to hear the Lord's instruction? In other words, are you actually denying the voice of the Lord so that you won't be held accountable for doing what He has asked you?

Give some thoughtful prayer to this today and make a heart adjustment where needed. Get your words and actions in line with His instructions and results. If you want His help and victory, you must do this by operating within the principles of Kingdom of God.

If you see that you have missed it, repent and turn from that path. Go back and receive the instructions He has brought you in the past and begin doing them. If He has placed someone in your life to instruct in the Word, then listen and do what they show you in the Word! Then, but only then, will you be able to move past current stumbling blocks into a future of victory, blessing, and harvest!

THE PICTURE OF HEALTH®
DAILY POWER PLAN™
Day 50

Acts 28:27 (KJV)

> For the heart of this people is waxed gross, and their ears are dull of hearing, and their eyes have they closed; lest they should see with their eyes, and hear with their ears, and understand with their heart, and should be converted, and I should heal them.

Selah (pause and reflect)

For several years now the Lord has had me on a continual journey into His Word. As I grow, mature, and become more and more obedient to listen, He continues to reveal to my understanding (through His Word) the undeniable *union* and *communion* between our Spirit, Soul, and Body. It is and has been the most amazing journey, part of which I hope to give you a taste of today with more in the days to come.

Just a few days ago, my pastor took me to the verse of scripture above in Acts 28. As my pastor spoke about the verse, once again the Lord unfolded a wonderful "nugget" regarding this fascinating relationship between the spiritual, the intellectual, and the physical man.

What caught my heart's attention were the particular effects listed in verse 27: "the heart of this people is waxed gross, and their ears are dull of hearing, and their eyes have they closed". The Lord opened my eyes of my understanding so that I saw in this passage, the explanation for three sets of physical symptoms, or more accurately stated, three common major diseases!

Look: 1) waxed hearts: atherosclerosis - hardening of the arteries (heart disease), 2) dull hearing: hearing loss (like Meniere's disease), and 3) closed eyes: cataracts, macular degeneration, and possibly presbyopia.

In the natural, all three of those categories are caused in great part by damage due to elevated homocysteine levels in the body. If you have taken The Picture of Health® Series 1, we learn that homocysteine is a natural part of the body's system which should be broken down into anti-inflammatory substances. Under certain conditions of the body (which you can learn about in class[1]), the homocysteine does not break down, as it should. When left as homocysteine, it becomes a destroyer in the body, especially to epithelial and endothelial tissue. That's right, tie it back to the scripture and you accurately find that this tissue is found in the arteries and vessels to the **heart, inner ear areas, and eyes!** (Also found in the reproductive areas and other organs, including the skin, but we'll save that for later!)

Okay, so that may not be exciting to you yet, perhaps you don't even see it yet, but I believe that God will reveal this to those *who will* see, hear, and receive. **It is about the connection.** If you will see the connection, you can receive the answer, *both spiritually and physically, to all disease.*

Oh... this is too big for one day's reading to hold! Here's what we will do: take this much - a teaspoon full we'll say - and pray about it. If you truly desire to see what the Lord is teaching - how to be healthy in every way - then confess to the Lord that you desire to see, to hear, and to receive His truth in your heart. Ask Him to open the eyes of your understanding as we study this out that we will *not* be those who are deaf, blind, and diseased. When we seek Him *to be* the ones who *do* understand, who *do turn* to Him, and who *do receive* His healing, we shall be.

If you need help praying this out, go in your Bible to Psalm 119: 65-73 and pray it aloud. Even better, if you can take the time, read the whole Psalm 119 at least once this week. I'll be praying it with you! And we will pick it up here and continue tomorrow!

THE PICTURE OF HEALTH®
DAILY POWER PLAN™

Day 51

Matthew 13:15 (NIV)

> For this people's heart has become
> calloused; they hardly hear with their ears,
> and they have closed their eyes. Otherwise
> they might see with their eyes, hear with
> their ears, understand with their hearts and
> turn, and I would heal them.

> *<u>Selah (pause and reflect)</u>*

Oh how my heart longs for you to see the opportunity the Lord is bringing to one or more of you, today! I truly believe He is inviting us to receive something very precious - something that will change our lives, perhaps even save our lives. I ask you to believe with me that I will be enabled by Him to express what He has put in my heart for you.

We left off yesterday in prayer that we would each see, hear, and receive His truth in our hearts and that we would turn to Him and be healed. So let's pick up there today, believing the answer to that prayer is manifest in us, thereby expecting that we will receive revelation of His truth from the Word of God.

Our scripture today from Matthew has the same text that we looked at yesterday in Acts Chapter 28. Since the original text is from Isaiah Chapter 6, this makes three places so far in the Word that we see this statement from the Lord. If you were with me yesterday, we saw that these verses are not only addressing a spiritual condition of one's heart, but that these verses may also convey wisdom to us about three major areas of disease in the physical body. (This is supported by or evidenced by the Lord's statement, "Otherwise...I would *heal* them".) But where is *"the connection"* and *what does it mean to our health*?

In Mark 8:17, Jesus asked his disciples, "Do you still not see or understand? Are your hearts hardened?" In this scripture He shows us that the hardened heart is linked with not hearing, seeing, or understanding. But I also believe that the Lord is bringing revelation to us through all these passages as to how *the dullness of a spiritually hardened heart causes a physically hardened heart as well.*

If we look just a little earlier in Acts Chapter 28, we uncover *the root: Why were their hearts hardened?* Acts 28:24 says: (italics mine)

> And some *believed* the things which were spoken, and some *believed not.*

I learned that this word for believed (peitho {pi'-tho} in the Greek) means *persuaded* or *un-persuadable*. And the Word goes on to tell us in verse 26, "...Go unto this people (**the un-persuadable people**), and say, Hearing ye shall hear, and shall not understand; and seeing ye shall see, and not perceive...".

So...the reason these people *didn't understand* was because they first chose to be un-persuadable of God's truth.

Did you get that? They were un-persuadable, *not* ignorant. This has to mean that the Lord brought revelation to the people about something (anything) and *they did not want to or choose to receive it from Him!* They chose not to believe it. They chose to operate as if the Lord never brought it to their attention. They refused to listen.

That's right! What a great memory you have! We did study rejecting His knowledge just a few weeks ago in Luke 8:18 and Hosea 4:6. And, I found this verse in 2 Thessalonians 2:10 (NLT) to add to our previous study: (Italics mine.)

> He (the evil one) will use every kind of wicked deception to fool those who are on their way to destruction ***because they refuse to believe the truth*** *that would save them.*

The new light or revelation in this is that *the result (<u>on the way to destruction</u>) was a* **hardened heart**.

That is where "the connection" lies…at the hardened heart and *why* it was hardened. Tomorrow we will tie it all back in with our discussion of the natural disease process and how these two pieces of knowledge connect in life-giving revelation. For tonight, I leave you with Psalm 95:7-8:

> **For he is our God and we are the people of his pasture, the flock under his care. Today, if you hear his voice, do not harden your hearts.**

THE PICTURE OF HEALTH®
DAILY POWER PLAN™
Day 52

Genesis 1:26-27 (AMP)

> God said, Let Us [Father, Son, and Holy Spirit] make mankind in Our image, after Our likeness, and let them have complete authority over the fish of the sea, the birds of the air, the [tame] beasts, and over all of the earth, and over everything that creeps upon the earth. So God created man in His own image, in the image and likeness of God He created him; male and female He created them.

Selah (pause and reflect)

You may recall that I said a couple of days ago that the reason to be excited was because this piece of revelation we are exploring is all about "the connection". So, what is it?

Yesterday's closing thoughts were, "But the new light in this is that the result (on the way to destruction) was a hardened heart." That is where "the connection" lies - at the hardened heart and why it was hardened. Let's tie it all back in now with our discussion of the natural disease process and how these two pieces of knowledge connect in life-giving revelation.

The connection actually is the inseparable union and communion between our Spirit, Soul, and Body. The Lord tells us in Genesis 1:26-27 that we are made in His image. Our three parts, like His three parts (Father, Son, and Holy

Spirit) are three-in-one, all unique but never functioning completely independent of one another. To the degree we understand this, we can better see in the Word answers as to why we sometimes fail to walk in the full victory He purchased for us. This applies particularly to the victory He desires for us now, in this life in the natural world, and specifically in the realm of our physical health!

The Greek word for this "communion" of Spirit, Soul, and Body is koinonia (koy-nohn-ee'-ah). It means fellowship, joint participation, and intercourse. It expresses the characteristic of *intimacy*. The verses we have been studying this week are perfect examples of how this communion, this intercourse and joint-participation, causes action or activity in one area (Spirit, Soul, or Body) to always have an affect on the other two areas.

We learned from all the verses we looked at that a hardened heart is a *result of* refusing to hear His voice, a result of closing your eyes to His wisdom, and a result of one's choice to turn away and remain un-believing, un-persuadable. So we have an action in the Soul (your mind, will, and emotions) that causes a result in the Spirit. Let me say it again this way: a hardened heart, which is *a spiritual condition* toward God, *is a result of* an action in our Soul (*rejecting God's knowledge or instruction*).

There we have two of the three areas of our Spirit, Soul, and Body affected by the one action. Now, if we are made in His image with three parts, bound together in communion (joint-participation), there must be a result that occurs in the body as well. What is it?

The scripture teaches us that a hardened spiritual heart leads to destruction as a result of separation from the Lord's protection and provision (through rejecting His knowledge and teaching). <u>That is a definition of sin</u>. The Bible declares in Romans that the <u>wages</u> of (result or payment for) sin is *death*. So, **death is the result in the physical body**.

Now let's look at the medical implications of this. In the natural, we learned that elevated homocysteine levels harden the heart, dull the hearing, and blind the eyes. *Can you see it?* These are the <u>same three results</u> in the Spirit as in the Body!

What I am saying is, in the light of these many scriptures we have looked at, perhaps the Lord has tried to give us knowledge and correction in some area and we rejected it or closed our eyes and pretended not to hear Him. That issue, whatever it is with Him, is sin (for which the wages is death) that has the power to literally have resulted in the physical body as a hardened heart, dull hearing, or blind eyes.

Still not persuaded? We can actually trace the path scientifically in the natural body. Watch this:

Disobedience and rebellion is sin. Destroying the temple of God is sin. Worry is sin. Lying is sin. Promiscuity is sin. Whatever it is you are doing that is in conflict with God's Word, it is sin. Now, having established that, you fill in the blank with the name of that sin every time you see the word "sin" in this next illustration of how a spiritual action causes a physical ailment or disease. Ready?

It is proven by medical research and experience that stress taxes the body and uses up all your body's reserves (minerals, vitamins, energy). When you don't have adequate reserves available, you can't fight off inflammation, destruction, and disease. When you have no mineral and vitamin reserves, one result is that the homocysteine in the body does not break down, as it should into anti-inflammatories. Instead, it remains in the blood stream and circulates causing damage to arteries and other body tissues. The body attempts to repair that damage by plaquing up the arteries with cholesterol. The plaque in the arteries eventually causes the condition of hardening...the hardened heart manifest in the physical body; the damage in the ear...loss of hearing; the damage to the vessels of the eyes...blind eyes.

It is a spiritual principle acted on by choice in the soul with result in the body. It may be that He tried to speak with us about our natural choices in the body and we put it off or didn't want to hear Him. Or perhaps He tried to teach us how to care for temple and we rejected the instruction. Or, really, it could be whatever issue He has been trying to instruct and enlighten any of us in. Whatever it is, it is rebellion. And the result is destruction.

And here's another powerful illustration dealing with damage to the brain producing loss of memory and understanding (such as happens with Alzheimer's). How do we get that?

Sin causes separation from God and the love of God. Sin opens the door for fear. Fear-based living is manifest as stress in our lives. It is a medical truth that stress uses up our body's reserves of the mineral zinc at alarming rates. How does that tie in and why is that important?

Zinc is the intelligence mineral - a protector of the brain. Without zinc, one gradually loses good brain function. In fact, a research study published in *Neurology*, January 25, 2005 states "persons prone to distress were 2.4 times more likely to develop Alzheimer's disease than persons not distress prone"!

Need more proof? Zinc is also connected with taste and smell. Research suggests that it is common for Alzheimer's patients to lose their taste and smell about two years before other symptoms are evident!

I am telling you, beloved, the Lord is ever surrounding us with knowledge to lead us from the way of destruction if we will only listen!

The Word says *turn*...and He will heal you!

So, where does that leave us? With great revelation! Disease is no longer some horrible mystery that we have no say about! If there is a problem in the physical body, you need to check your heart! Ask the Lord what He has tried or is trying to show you, repent for rejecting His instruction, and *do* whatever it is He has asked, even if it doesn't seem connected to the physical symptoms! Then, praise the Lord and be persuaded of your recovery!

THE PICTURE OF HEALTH®
DAILY POWER PLAN™
Day 53

Daniel 1:15 (NIV)

> At the end of the ten days they looked healthier and better nourished than any of the young men who ate the royal food.

Selah (pause and reflect)

Wow! How did they do it?

These four youths were "guests" in a place of extravagant temptation in terms of rich foods and luxuries. Because they were in captivity in a foreign land, it is correct to say that they were under a good amount of emotional and physical stress. In our lives, most would say that these boys had plenty of good excuses for not honoring God in their bodies.

If you check earlier in this chapter you will see that Daniel resolved not to defile himself with the king's temptations, including the "rich meat and dainties". Later we see that he resolved not to let anything about his captivity defile his walk with God. These four boys are quite a good study. Let's just stick with one topic for today:

Daniel determined not to make excuses. At all costs, he determined not to be defiled. The Bible tells us that he requested of his jailer,

> "Please test your servants for ten days: Give us nothing but vegetables to eat and water to drink. Then compare our appearance with

> that of the young men who eat the royal food, and treat your servants in accordance with what you see." So he agreed to this and tested them for ten days. (Daniel 1:13-14)

How many of you ask to be tested when you are under stress? Here is the result: At the end of the ten days they looked healthier and better nourished than any other! The refusal to make excuses and the commitment to their relationship with God provided unmatched results in just ten days!

What was at work here that perhaps you haven't experienced? It wasn't just a diet that made these boys "the picture of health". It was the application of the Biblical principle of fasting. Not dieting mind you which is reducing or abstaining from food(s) to affect just the physical body, but true Biblical *fasting*.

Let's look at the difference and perhaps many of you will get wisdom and understanding as to why your attempts at health or physical improvement have failed thus far.

First, Daniel determined in his heart that he would bring the body into submission and to keep the spirit and soul undefiled from the customs of the new world around them. He wasn't merely eating differently. <u>He abstained from selected items for a specific purpose and did so unto God.</u>

By his actions and submission to God and the results thereof, Daniel was proclaiming to his captors, "My God, the Almighty God, is different than your gods. I reverence Him for He is Holy. My choices are different from the pagan world around me because of who He is and how I reverence Him."

If you read further in Daniel, one will see this bears out in the continued hand of God upon Daniel and his companions. I believe Daniel's decision to fast was a huge contributor to the spiritual strength we later see in all of these young men.

So, how does one method of abstinence (dieting) produce sickness and death and another method (fasting unto the Lord) produce strength and health?

In the natural, dieting subtracts from one's health. Typically, people force the body into starvation to reduce weight. Perhaps they abstain from fats in an attempt to influence a change in cholesterol levels. Either way, the abstinence is about food, not God. Another way to say that would be that abstinence from food by dieting is separate from your relationship with God. That which is separate from God is what? Diets result in the body's scavenging muscle and bone for survival rather than burning excess fat and eliminating toxic waste.

In sharp contrast, the entry for "fasting" in *Vine's Expository Dictionary* states,

"Christ taught the need of purity and simplicity of motive. The answers of Christ to the questions of the disciples of John and of the Pharisees reveal His whole purpose and method." "What He taught was suitable *to the change of character and purpose which He designed for His disciples*." (Emphasis added.)

Fasting is not so much about denying yourself as it is about not defiling yourself.

The Lord knows the intent of your heart. Your true motive is not disguised from His eyes. If you are dieting and calling it a fast, He knows. So also does the destroyer who is waiting for just such an opportunity to devour you. But if you are truly being led by the Lord to fast from something for the strengthening of your spirit and your body, then your time will be consecrated unto the Lord and the destroyer will have no opportunity to harm you.

Enter in first by prayer, and continue by replacing whatever is laid aside for the time of the fast with time spent in the Lord. Allow yourself time to draw nearer to God and focus on His desires for your life and your body. If you keep these things in mind and be Spirit-led, you, like Daniel, will come out stronger, not weaker, a true testimony to the Lord!

THE PICTURE OF HEALTH®
DAILY POWER PLAN™
Day 54

1 John 2:16 (NLT)

> For the world offers only the lust for physical pleasure, the lust for everything we see, and pride in our possessions. These are not from the Father. They are from this evil world.

<u>*Selah (pause and reflect)*</u>

Have you ever noticed? When we begin to make changes to improve the way we care for the temple of God, sometimes the body or the flesh tries to rebel?

See, the body used to be of the world, knew the world, and liked the pleasures of the world. However, when you became "In Christ" by accepting Him as your Lord and Savior, you were born-again of the Spirit on the inside and redeemed from the death of this world and its worldly lusts. But, when you begin to walk in that redemption inside, sometimes the body, the outside, is tempted to return to the old ways.

This attempt at rebellion is the same with any habit or pattern of behavior; they must be brought into submission of the new man. The Word tells us in Romans 12:2 (NIV) <u>*how*</u> we change from the old life of destruction and death to the new life in the Spirit:

> Do not conform any longer to the pattern of this world, but be transformed by the

renewing of your mind. Then you will be
able to test and approve what God's will
is–his good, pleasing and perfect will.

The Word of God also tells us in 1 Timothy 6:17 that God richly provides us with everything to enjoy! Walking in the fullness of the love of God puts all good things at our disposal - to enjoy! Psalm 103:5 (KJV) even tells us that it is the Lord "who satisfieth thy mouth with *good things*; *so that* thy youth is renewed like the eagle's". (Emphasis mine.)

In Christ, you are not at all deprived and never will be again.

I saw a great illustration of this over the weekend. Take a piece of paper and mark a period (a small black dot) in the middle of the paper. Now, look at the paper and tell me what you see. You see a black dot. But that is not really all that you see. Don't you also see a large expanse of white paper? There is a *greater* amount of white on the paper than there is of the black dot.

Beloved, the changes that produce health are not about what we can't have. It is about what we can and do have in Christ and if we choose to partake of it! It is about the *greater*. Greater than all the things of the world are what we have and enjoy in Christ!

The Word says, "Greater is He that is in you than he that is in the world." I discussed this with a friend just yesterday. We agreed that people would never resist His Way for our live if we only knew His character. When you *know* Him, you have no difficulty believing that what He has for us is greater that we anything can ask, think, or imagine! Why would anyone resist following that?

God gives you richly all good things to enjoy. He fills your mouth with good things so that your youth is renewed like the eagle!

"Bless the Lord! Bless the Lord, O my soul and forget not all His benefits!"

THE PICTURE OF HEALTH®
DAILY POWER PLAN™
Day 55

Mark 7:15 (NLT)

> You are not defiled by what you eat; you are defiled by what you say and do!

Selah (pause and reflect)

We've just been examining in recent days "the connection", the communion of our Spirit, Soul, and Body as made in the image of God. We have also been studying the pull of the world and the temptation to be defiled by its lusts. These temptations are the weapons of the enemy. The Bible clearly identifies for us the only methods the enemy has to tempt us: (parenthesis added for identification)

> For all that is in the world, the lust of the flesh *(body)*, and the lust of the eyes *(soul)*, and the pride of life *(spirit)*, is not of the Father, but is of the world. 1 John 2:16 (KJV)

Note the words: "of the world." The Word says in 1 Corinthians 2:12 (NIV) that, "We have not received the spirit of the world but the Spirit who is from God, that we may understand what God has freely given us." And Jesus said it this way in Mark 7 (NLT) beginning in verse 14,

> "…All of you listen," he said, "and try to understand. You are not defiled by what you eat; you are defiled by what you say

and do!" then later the disciples asked him what he meant and Jesus replied, "Don't you understand either?" he asked. "Can't you see that what you eat won't defile you? Food doesn't come in contact with your heart, but only passes through the stomach and then comes out again." (By saying this, he showed that every kind of food is acceptable.) And then he added, "It is the thought-life that defiles you."

Real victory over the lusts of the world comes when you understand and submit to the knowledge that the battle for the flesh is won in the Spirit and manifest through the actions of the Soul.

For example, in *The Picture of Health®* classes, people frequently ask for a more structured eating plan. They don't want to be responsible for making choices, "just tell me what to eat". What they are really wanting is a *diet*. 1 Timothy 4 (NIV) considers diets this way:

> The Spirit clearly says that in later times some will abandon the faith and follow deceiving spirits and things taught by demons.
>
> Such teachings come through hypocritical liars, whose consciences have been seared as with a hot iron. They forbid people to marry and order them to abstain from certain foods, which God created to be received with thanksgiving by those who believe and who know the truth.
>
> For everything God created is good, and nothing is to be rejected if it is received with

> thanksgiving, because it is consecrated by
> the word of God and prayer.

Diets are rooted in wrong thinking patterns that ultimately end up in ruin. So, we have been led by the Lord not to give in to that thinking pattern and not to comply with requests that will hold people in bondage.

The world has trained people to think that we can control our bodies better if we have some regulations to follow. But see, that is why they are in the class to begin with... suffering from dis-ease caused by following the world's pattern, which has obviously not worked for them so far and never will for any length of time! One more diet will not achieve what they are really seeking after.

Jesus said in the verse above, "It is your thought life that defiles you." Your thought life dictates the way you think about your body, your health, what is required to achieve that health, and the biggie: the true definition of what "the picture of health" really is.

Many people think a certain look or weight shows one's health. Wrong. Others define health as the absence of dis-ease. And that is getting warmer although not quite all the way there. Divine health as purchased for us on the cross is much more than appearance of health in the physical.

I believe the definition we are looking for is not diet and is not even health. What we are truly seeking is:

> **Shalom** – (shalowm {shaw-lome'} or shalom {shaw-lome}) Completeness, soundness, welfare, health, prosperity, peace, contentment, nothing missing, nothing broken, friendship with God in covenant relationship.

You will never find divine health in a set of laws.

You will find it in your covenant with God.

When the enemy of your soul comes to tempt you with the lusts of the eyes, the lusts of the flesh, or the pride of life (rebellion), what will you do?

Will you live mastered by the world's deception and destruction for the rest of your life just to satisfy the cravings of your carnal nature and flesh?

Or, will you be transformed by the renewing of your mind that you may understand what God in His infinite goodness has freely given us? The decision, the choice, is yours to make.

"Choose you this day whom ye will serve;

whether the gods which your fathers served that [were] on the other side of the flood,

or the gods of the Amorites, in whose land ye dwell:

but as for me and my house, we will serve the LORD."

Joshua 24:15 (KJV)

Now and forever, **I pray for you, "Shalom"**.

THE PICTURE OF HEALTH®
DAILY POWER PLAN™
Day 56

Hebrews 8:5-7 (New International Version)

> They serve at a sanctuary that is a copy and shadow of what is in heaven. This is why Moses was warned when he was about to build the tabernacle: "See to it that you make everything according to the pattern shown you on the mountain."
>
> But the ministry Jesus has received is as superior to theirs as the covenant of which he is mediator is superior to the old one, and it is founded on better promises.
>
> For if there had been nothing wrong with that first covenant, no place would have been sought for another.

Selah (pause and reflect)

"What is wrong with dieting anyway?" "What about xyz diet, that's not really bad for us, is it?" "Isn't this plan the same as xyz diet? My friend lost weight on that diet and they eat 1 cup of vegetables per day. That sounds the same to me." "How about the cabbage diet - that is a vegetable, isn't it? Isn't that healthy?"

I will repeat myself from yesterday,

> *You will never find divine health in a set of laws.*
>
> *You will find it in your covenant with God.*

Beloved, it is true that diets are dangerous to your physical health. Their unbalanced nutritional structure alone makes them damaging to the body. But more than that, they are damaging to your spiritual health and to your soul's emotional and mental health.

The old covenant was based on law and brought about guilt, punishment, and condemnation. That is the very essence of dieting. Dieting and the desire to diet make you a slave again to the law, to guilt, to condemnation, and ultimately to failure.

The old covenant was only a shadow of the glorious new one to come through Christ. The scripture says that the new covenant is "far superior to the old one". Our covenant is a covenant of grace and freedom.

So why do people still diet? <u>Because it takes more self-control to walk in freedom than it does to follow rules.</u> But! Self-control is the fruit of the Holy Spirit! If you walk in the spirit, you have the power of self-control.

When one learns to rest in the covenant we have through Christ and begins to renew the mind through the Word of God, we begin to understand who we really are in Christ and the place our body holds in the Kingdom of God. With that new understanding, great freedom comes. With the freedom found in the covenant also comes power from the Holy Spirit and victory through the Blood of Christ.

Philippians 4:13 (KJV) tells me, "I can do all things through Christ which strengtheneth me." That means I no longer have to live by a diet. Because I am in Christ and He is in me, I have the strength to make choices in my physical body that produce health *and* the strength to walk them out *as* I choose to!

Dieting and diet mentalities rob you of that freedom and the accompanying strength. If you truly want victory, whether it is over too much weight, or too little, or too high cholesterol, or cancer, or whatever...there is only one way to that victory. What is that way? Jesus answered that question in John 4:16 (NIV):

"I am the way and the truth and the life.

No one comes to the Father except through me."

The way, the truth, and the life apply to *every aspect* of your walk...including your physical health. I mean, just read it...*the way* to walk in health, *the truth* of how that can happen...how to do it, *the life* your physical body needs.

Victory will never be found in *any* diet ever written.

Victory is found in your covenant through Christ and the power of the Holy Spirit.

The turning point between death, diets, and disease is the moment you get the revelation that the law brings bondage and the new covenant brings freedom and victory.

Earlier this year I heard someone say, "Christianity is not a behavior modification program. Christianity is a heart transformation program." How true!

When you decide to turn to the covenant for your answers, every answer, you will walk in the fullness of your redemption through Christ. Then, beloved, you will surely taste and see that the Lord is good. When you truly know Him, you never desire to return to the bondage of the law again!

There is an anointing working right now where you are for that freedom. The Word tells us that signs and wonders will follow the preaching and teaching of the Word. My voice may not be heard where you are right now, but the Voice of the Lord is heard through His Word. That means that signs and wonders shall confirm that Word.

If you need healing in your body, freedom in your soul, and/or the fruit of self-control by the power of the Holy Spirit, *receive it now*. Repent of following the world's way of dieting and by faith lay hold of His benefits through your covenant in Christ. Take that step of faith and declare His Word aloud:

"I have been set free from the law of sin and death. I am a new creation in Christ, made in the image of the Most High God! His Spirit right now lives in me and is ever producing life and health in every part of my spirit, soul, and body. I will never again allow myself to be made a slave to bondage. It is for freedom I have been made free!"

Glory to God! I know in my spirit that for all who will believe the Word of God, signs and wonders and healing miracles are taking place in their lives today. I know because His Word never returns void but accomplishes that for which it was sent. I know because He is faithful to do above all that we could ask, think, or imagine! And I also know because He has done it in me.

If you prayed today, believe Him and thank Him for it! Rejoice in it! This is no small victory! You are free beloved. You are finally free! Now walk it out with Him daily, spending time in the Word and yielding to the fruit of the Spirit in your life.

THE PICTURE OF HEALTH®
DAILY POWER PLAN™
Day 57

Proverbs 4:20-22 (NKJV)

My son, give attention to my words;

Incline your ear to my sayings.

Do not let them depart from your eyes;

Keep them in the midst of your heart;

For they *are* life to those who find them,

And health to all their flesh.

Selah (pause and reflect)

Nothing I can say about diets or the dangers of dieting can make it any more plain than the Lord has in today's scripture. *The Word of God* is <u>health</u> <u>and</u> <u>life</u> *to all your flesh.*

It would have to flat-out rebellion to allow the dieting mindset to remain after reading this verse. You see, friends, the Lord has just revealed to us THE WAY to have life and health in our whole body...and it is not by dieting!

With such a clear Word and a better covenant, what an enormous tragedy it is then that many people still stubbornly live in darkness, dying early, short of their purpose, burned out and used up before their full age because they reject this knowledge!

Have you ever noticed that sometimes the Word of God rises up in you in so much faith that it is like a fire shut up in your bones? Well, beloved, I for one think that the enemy of our soul has kept the body of Christ in deception about this truth for way too long!

And while I am inspired to be so bold, I will also say that too many of us have let our carnal nature keep us in denial to the voice of God!

God *is* interested in the condition of your physical body! It is time for us to wakeup, bring our flesh into submission to the Spirit, and rebuke the devourer of our health!

All of the scriptures we have studied so far indicate that Christians fail to live in health for one of three reasons: lack of faith, lack of knowledge, or rebellion (disobedience) against the Word of God.

Let us be those who are doers of the Word. Let us heed what the Lord is so graciously bringing to us day by day. Let us take this Word to heart and apply our faith in obedience so that we are not among the perishing any longer! Let us receive revelation from God's Word about health and life. And let us allow the power of God to transform us spirit, soul, and body!

THE PICTURE OF HEALTH®
DAILY POWER PLAN™
Day 58

1 John 5:4 (AMP)

> For whatever is born of God is victorious over the world; and this is the victory that conquers the world, even our faith.

Selah (pause and reflect)

I marvel at how the Lord is leading us! "This is the victory that conquers (overcomes) the world"! I believe the Lord is showing us that there is greater meaning, greater depth to this scripture than we have seen before.

This morning, even after reading this verse so many times before, I was lifted up to a higher place of revelation. This has always been a verse of encouragement, but today as I read it, I realized that, for believers in Christ, <u>we are the "whosoever born of God"</u>.

Beloved, we have the victory in all things - both now and forever more. From the greatest things in life to the most basic things (like our health walk), we *are* conquerors. Romans 8:37 (AMP) says it this way: (emphasis added)

> Yet *amid all these things* we are more than conquerors and gain a surpassing victory through Him Who loved us.

Yes, I have mentally known that for some time. But today I looked at it in new light…not just a phrase learned as children long ago in Sunday school. No, today's revelation is a *rhema* Word, a revelation from God that I am truly made by Him more than a conqueror over what I face today.

What does that mean? It is time to stop settling for less than God's best! It means that not only can we do all things through Christ, which strengthens us, but also we are victorious over the world!

Now, wait…before you go putting on your church face and agree too quickly, you better give this some serious thought. I am speaking very plainly about natural things, things that we've just lost our excuses for doing. (Ouch!)

This tells us that we <u>are</u> (as in *already*) victorious over disease, illness, eating compulsions, aging, bad attitudes, griping, complaining…should I go on? We aren't about to be conquerors. We already are. Conquerors always win; it is the very definition of the word.

If we are conquerors, then let us be about acting in the confidence that would bring to us!

Begin to renew your mind with these powerful words, deliberately putting them into action in your lives. Speak out the complete victory that He provided for us! Take this Word and each of you fill in the blank with whatever challenges you today. Make the decision to release the things that are holding you back and embrace the victory! Today, we walk as conquerors!

THE PICTURE OF HEALTH® DAILY POWER PLAN™

Day 59

Isaiah 46:4 (NLT)

> I will be your God throughout your lifetime—until your hair is white with age. I made you, and I will care for you. I will carry you along and save you.

Selah (pause and reflect)

Today let's take a look at another aspect of God's character and love for us. Actually, it is the underlying reason we are over-comers. It is because He is the Lord our rescuer, our deliverer, in whom we can place our faith and draw the courage to face daily challenges.

The verse for today from the Word of God expresses His great love and His desire to protect us. This is much like the love I feel for my own children.

Before we go on, I think we should stop here and just read it again out loud a couple of times. Feel the great depths of His words to you, to each one of us: He says,

"I *made* you, and I will *care for you*. I will *carry you* along and *save* you."

The Greek word used here for "save" is "natsal {nawtsal'}". This word means to deliver, to rescue, to, literally, snatch you out (of peril). Did you know that this word is used in the King James Version *over 200 times* in reference to the Lord rescuing, saving, and delivering you and me, His beloved, from harm and from the enemy?

Wow. At least 200 times He says that *to me*.

The Word says in Isaiah 35,

> With this news, strengthen those who have tired hands, and encourage those who have weak knees. Say to those who are afraid, "Be strong, and do not fear, for your God is coming to destroy your enemies. He is coming to save you." And when he comes, he will open the eyes of the blind and unstop the ears of the deaf. The lame will leap like a deer, and those who cannot speak will shout and sing!

Not only does He want us to know that He will deliver us, but He desires us to encourage one another with this truth. Why? The verse from Isaiah is just one of many that answer that: so that <u>by faith in Him we will be healed</u>!

Look at all the diseases He lists there: arthritis, failing knees, blindness or vision loss, deafness or hearing loss, walking problems, and voice or speech problems. My goodness! What else could we list? Passages in Jeremiah tell of deliverance from torment, from enemies, from cruelty, from the world's ways. Like I said, over 200 times He speaks that He is our deliverer, our rescuer!

Why do I bring this out today? Because we face challenges as we walk in the Word to gain understanding about our bodies and our health, challenges which are directly related, like cravings of the flesh, habits that need to be changed, exercise that needs to be started, etc. We also face indirect challenges, like bad days where stress tempts us to reach for the wrong things to ease our anxiety. And there are challenges like busy schedules which position us to grab easy-to-eat food but food that doesn't nourish us or ugly people who get on your nerves and give you an excuse to harbor anger or un-forgiveness, which rots your body. You know… challenges.

Don't give in to defeat and reach for food or drink as your comfort. Reach for the rescuer of our Spirit, Soul, and Body! Psalms 25:15 says He will deliver you from that which ensnares you. In Jeremiah 1:19 (KJV), it is written:

"For I AM with thee, saith the LORD, to deliver thee."

Whatever the challenge - weight, pain, cancer, heart disease, emotional turmoil, boredom, or *anything* else, if you turn to Him today, He will deliver you and bring you through!

THE PICTURE OF HEALTH®
DAILY POWER PLAN™
Day 60

Luke 5:25 (AMP)

> And instantly [the man] stood up before them and picked up what he had been lying on and went away to his house, recognizing and praising and thanking God.

Selah (pause and reflect)

Conquerors! Overcomers! It is who we have been made to be! The Word of God tells us in Revelation 12:11 (AMP) that **"they have overcome (conquered) him by means of the blood of the Lamb and by the utterance of their testimony,** for they did not love and cling to life even when faced with death [holding their lives cheap till they had to die for their witnessing]." (Emphasis added.)

According to the scripture, the Blood of the Lamb (Christ) and the word of their testimony are the two characteristics necessary for the conqueror's success. Today, I'd like to examine *"the utterance (or the word) of their testimony."*

What is that: "your testimony"? If you are to overcome and conquer **by** the Blood and your testimony, it is pretty important that you understand what that is, right?

Well, right off you might think that your testimony is the story of how you came to know the Lord as your Savior. That is a common definition for your testimony. And what a glorious day, yes indeed! It is the greatest miracle of all!

But, I want to challenge you to go beyond that day. Do others around you know what God has done in your life *lately*? Does your life *still* draw others to the light and passion they see in you?

People are hungry for victory. They desperately want hope for what they are facing *right now*. They want to find who it is that has overcome and ask them to tell their "testimony" of how it happened.

If we look at examples in the Word, we begin to see a pattern common to the "over-comers". I found at least four recurrent steps in this pattern: 1) the person(s) <u>received</u> instruction from the Lord by faith, 2) they did what the Lord told them to <u>do</u>, 3) they <u>shared</u> that with and in front of others, and 4) they <u>give praise and thanks to the Lord.</u>

We see this pattern in Luke 17:11-19 (AMP), where verse 15 says, "…then one of them, upon seeing that he was cured, turned back, recognizing and thanking and praising God with a loud voice;" Jesus had told ten lepers to go show themselves to the priest and on their way, they were cleansed. So they all received instruction, went as Jesus instructed, but only one turned back, testified loudly so that others could hear and know, and returned to praise God and give thanks to the Lord.

Luke 5:25-26, our scripture text for today reads this way in the New International Version, "And immediately, as everyone watched, the man jumped to his feet, picked up his mat, and went home praising God." Then, this is what I am getting at today, the Word goes on to say,

> Everyone was gripped with great wonder and awe. And they praised God, saying over and over again; "We have seen amazing things today."

"As everyone watched..." they were gripped with great wonder and awe, praising God!

If you are reading this today, I want you to know that this whole book is me, jumping up before you and praising the Lord, sharing with you what He has done and is doing in my life. In fact, everything to do with <u>*The Picture of Health*</u> is our testimony to the power of God at work in our lives, our family, our finances, and our health, and in every area. And you know what? I'm not ashamed of that.

Like the man from our text, *I have been made whole* not only for my own sake, but also for your sake and *for His glory*! It is my testimony! So, I praise the Lord openly, loudly, for what He has done! I boast in it like Paul. Not in my ability or works, but in my weaknesses, He is magnified for making me a conqueror! Yes, that's right…in my weakness He is being magnified!

See, my friends, I spent most of the first thirty years of my life trying to be strong and conquer the world. And, because I am not *designed* to do so in my own strength, my life fell completely apart under the constant pressure of attaining perfection.

But Oh! Glory to God! The freedom that came when I surrendered the lordship of my life to Him and learned to walk in His (immeasurable) strength instead! Now, *in weakness I am being perfected*…spiritually, mentally, emotionally, and physically. So, I rejoice that He has restored me in all things that are good!

How could I not tell of His wonders?

And, beloved, some of those wonders are <u>you</u>! Each week I see His handiwork in your lives, in your physical bodies gaining strength and reclaiming health, and in your spiritual walk with Him...bringing newfound joy and radiance to your faces.

Many of you, just like me, have a testimony of daily victories large and small. For some of you, it is that He has reduced your insulin levels or has lowered LDL cholesterol levels. Some of you have overcome an eating disorder. Some of you have been healed of cancer by applying the wisdom and knowledge He has brought you. And I am certain there are many, many other examples.

"As everyone watched..."

You might be surprised at who it is that is watching you today. Isn't it time you stepped into your place as a conqueror and shared your testimony?

You have to power to ignite personal revival in your life and the lives of those around you. Testify of His faithfulness and mercy as He brings you out of death and destruction into health and life!

> Praise be to God who has made us a chosen race, a royal priesthood, a dedicated nation, God's own purchased, special people, ***that we may*** *set forth the wonderful deeds and display the virtues and perfections of Him Who called us out of darkness into His marvelous light!*
>
> 1 Peter 2:9 AMP (emphasis added)

THE PICTURE OF HEALTH®
DAILY POWER PLAN™
Day 61

Hebrews 9:14 (New International Version)

> How much more, then, will the blood of Christ, who through the eternal Spirit offered himself unblemished to God, cleanse our consciences from acts that lead to death, (or: from useless rituals) so that we may serve the living God!

<u>Selah (pause and reflect)</u>

In yesterday's walk, although we studied about our "testimony", we saw also that the Blood of Christ was one of two characteristics necessary for the conqueror's success. Let's pick that back up today.

The Blood of Christ, shed for us, is the entire reason we can have life and health at all. As we study the Blood of Christ, we will see the undeniable connection between true holiness and divine health.

Our recent devotionals have centered on the truth that we are *meant* to spend life ruling and reigning as *conquerors*, not as victims. Hebrews 9:14 tells us that it is by the Blood of the Lamb and the word of our testimony that we are equipped to conquer!

Today we see it is also the Blood of Christ that will cleanse our consciences from acts that lead to death, from useless rituals, so that we may serve God! That was good news to me. When I began this journey, I couldn't imagine how

I was going to ever renew my mind that was so full of dieting, rebellion, and independence. I was programmed nearly from birth by society to "bring home the bacon and fry it up too". I had a life of "useless rituals", including but not limited to dieting, that were slowly but surely stealing my health.

But the Lord is Jehovah Jireh! He is the Lord who sees ahead and provides! In this case, He provided the Blood of Christ to cleanse me from those acts that lead to death and the Word to tell me so! As I expressed my desire to walk in His truth so that I could serve Him more and be a greater testimony of His goodness, He came with the power to make it so…the power of the Blood of Christ. And He will for you as well.

1 Peter 2:5 (NIV) says:

> You also, like living stones, are being built into a spiritual house to be a holy priesthood, offering spiritual sacrifices acceptable to God through Jesus Christ.

Beloved, in these 100 days (and beyond), as we offer our lives as a spiritual sacrifice to Him, we are being built into His holy priesthood. "Being built" is the emphasis. Not building ourselves, but "being built" through Christ. Not by my blood, sweat, and tears, but quite literally ***by His***.

Let the Blood of Christ strengthen you today and give you courage! If you have faltered, let His Word empower you by the Blood to rededicate yourself. Even if you haven't faltered, take this opportunity to renew your commitment to do the things that produce a strong healthy you, remembering the purpose: (Ephesians 2:8-10 NIV)

For it is by grace you have been saved, through faith – and this not from yourself, it is the gift of God – not by works, so that no one can boast. For we are God's workmanship, created in Christ to do good works, which God prepared in advance for us to do.

THE PICTURE OF HEALTH®
DAILY POWER PLAN™
Day 62

Hebrews 7:25 (New International Version)

> Therefore he is able to save completely those who come to God through him, because he always lives to intercede for them.

Selah (pause and reflect

Everything about His life and death, even the very way in which he suffered made him able to *completely* save us. This is more of "the connection" the Lord keeps revealing to us through the Word.

Let's look at how he redeemed us spirit, soul, and body by the ways he suffered at the cross:

1) 'He was bruised (beaten) for our iniquities.' A bruise is below the surface, which is internal bleeding. This can be seen as payment for the internal sins in the *soul*.

2) 'By His stripes we were healed.' The stripes were where His skin was torn and bled from the violent whippings, seen as payment for sins in the *body*.

3) 'He was pierced for our transgressions.' Pierced through, where blood (carrying DNA generation to generation) and water (type of the spirit) flowed from his side. These can be seen as propitiation for all sins in all generations, a generational cleansing in the blood (actually capable of changing DNA)

and in the *spirit, all previous sin, all sin committed now, and all sin forever.*

Saved completely… Spirit, Soul, and Body

I know this may be a radical revelation for some of you, but don't take my word for it, look up all the many scriptures in the Word which link health in the body and the spirit. (You'll get a good start in the book of *Romans*.)

We can have victory <u>*in our physical body*</u> today because of how He suffered and died for us. The Lord wants you, and every believer to know that this redemptive victory in your physical body is yours, now and forever. He has cleansed (not covered, but cleansed!) you in His blood and washed your bodies with pure water. (Heb 10:22)

Why is this so important? SO THAT so that we may serve the living God! And, so that we don't waste one bit of the price He paid by not appropriating it into victory in our lives!

Yes we still live in a fallen world. And, yes, our bodies won't be fully glorified until He returns and catches us away. But his suffering did purchase for us divine health in this natural physical body. It is possible to live without disease. When your time is completed here, you can simply walk up to the mountain and go home to God.

I want to share a personal example of this powerful truth. My husband and I were visiting with my mother-in-law, Thera Pearson, on Mother's Day a few years ago. She was rejoicing that all her children and grandchildren knew the Lord and reflecting on how many years she had been without her husband, who had gone home before. She told us, "I am ready to go home now." One month later on Father's Day, she did just that.

Mom Pearson was healthy and lived alone to the night she went home. Knowing that all her loved ones are all saved and bound for heaven and after having lived a long and satisfying life on earth, she longed for His embrace. Evidently, she took a bath, laid across her bed, and woke up in His presence. If there is a more beautiful way to go home, I can't imagine it. We too can go home in just such glory.

Beloved friends, please let me tell you, the intents and objectives of the enemy today are still to steal, kill, and destroy. He wants to steal your health now so that you are useless to the kingdom and useless to the great commission. He wants to kill your physical body so that you cannot tell anyone else about Christ! He wants to destroy your witness and your life so that no one sees any victory in it! But...

There is the Blood of Christ! We won't be destroyed, and no longer will be content to let the enemy steal from us! No! That won't be us! He is bringing us into new revelation and knowledge in the Word every day! We will possess the victory, completely!

You should spend time today building yourself up in the truth about your body. Hold up your shield of faith to reject the enemy's attempts to destroy you! Remember that faith comes by hearing, and hearing the Word of God. Put the truth in your mouth as a sword against the enemy! Christ completely saved you, including the body.

According to the Word, we have complete salvation, healing, and deliverance! Determine today to honor the sacrifice by walking as a conqueror over your flesh! Lay hold of the blessing with vigor! Give thanks unto God, who according to the Word in 2 Corinthians 2:14 (KJV), ***always*** causes us to triumph in Christ and makes manifest the savour of his knowledge by us in ***every*** place!

THE PICTURE OF HEALTH®
DAILY POWER PLAN™
Day 63

2 Corinthians 3:18 (AMP)

> And all of us, as with unveiled face, [because we] continued to behold [in the Word of God] as in a mirror the glory of the Lord, are constantly being transfigured into His very own image in ever increasing splendor and from one degree of glory to another; [for this comes] from the Lord [Who is] the Spirit.

> ### *Selah (pause and reflect)*

Didn't I tell you? As we seek Him and give Him first place in our lives, He transfigures us into His image in ever-increasing splendor!

This word transfigured, means changed, or transformed. It comes from the Greek word "metamorphoo" {met-am-or-fo'-o}, where we get our word metamorphosis! This is the same word used to describe the remarkable change in Christ that was recorded in the Gospels. Here is the passage recorded in Luke 9:29-31, 34-35:

> As he was praying, the appearance of his face changed, and his clothes became as bright as a flash of lightning. Two men, Moses and Elijah, appeared in glorious splendor, talking with Jesus. They spoke about his departure, which he was about to bring to fulfillment at Jerusalem.

> While he was speaking, a cloud appeared and enveloped them, and they were afraid as they entered the cloud. A voice came from the cloud, saying, "This is my Son, whom I have chosen; listen to him."

I find it interesting that this transfiguration appears to be *part of Jesus' equipping for his purpose*. The transfiguration was not only internal or only spiritual. The Bible documents that the transformation caused a *physical change* in His appearance. The King James Version tells us "the fashion of his countenance was altered."

I also was captured by what followed in verses 34 and 35. The instruction to "listen to Him" further indicates that the transfiguration was a marking for purpose, a calling out, a choosing, and it was a confirmation of Christ's authority.

Why is this so exciting? Because God desires that experience for <u>*us*</u> as well! Armed with this knowledge, we should never again allow ourselves to get discouraged about physical problems, appearances, sickness, or disease! If we just return to the Word, we will see that He is the way to enact those desired physical changes and that *He desires to make those changes. He desires (even more than we do) that we be transformed* <u>in ever increasing splendor</u> from glory to glory <u>*so that*</u> our calling, the thing we have been chosen for from the beginning of time, can be fulfilled!

Romans 8:14 (KJV) says, "For as many as are led by the Spirit of God, they are the sons of God." Those of you, of us, who will be led by the Spirit of God, who will consecrate ourselves to Him and His desires for our lives, the Bible tells us...We are the sons of God. We are His chosen people, a royal priesthood!

<u>God wants you transfigured into His image!</u>

This is the great mystery being revealed to our generation! Yes! He wants to cause that to happen in your life and mine! And, the Bible says, *not* in the way of Moses, with a veiled face (lack of freedom and knowledge), "but we all, *with open face*...even as by the Spirit of the Lord."

Every day I realize more and more that this flesh, my body, is not mine to struggle with or against. He *wants* to do this in me! He wants my body to *glisten* from and in His transfiguration of my life and my countenance! WOW!

Can we even comprehend the length and depth and breadth of His love? Can we even imagine how *good* a body transformed by the power of God, made in His image will look? Or *how long that body could live* to witness of His love? Or *how far we could carry the gospel* with that much strength and health sustaining us?

That **is** His desire. Here is His request:

> "Behold, I stand at the door, and knock: if any man hear my voice, and open the door, I will come in to him, and will sup with him, and he with me.
>
> To him that overcometh will I grant to sit with me in my throne, even as I also overcame, and am set down with my Father in his throne." (Revelation 3:20-21 KJV)

Open the door.

THE PICTURE OF HEALTH®
DAILY POWER PLAN™
Day 64

Philippians 3:20-21 (NIV)

> But our citizenship is in heaven. And we eagerly await a Savior from there, the Lord Jesus Christ, who, by the power that enables him to bring everything under his control, will transform our lowly bodies so that they will be like his glorious body.

Selah (pause and reflect)

Think of it: We live in a time that no other generation has experienced. We have technology greater than any generation. We have resources discovered that no one has seen before. We can see farther and travel longer than any humans in history. But even more than all the natural advancements, we live in a time that is closer than any other to the Second Coming of Christ! Whenever that time is to be, we are closer than anyone has ever been.

If you talk to many people, you find that there is rising a great expectancy. Some with fear and some with excitement, but there is an intensity of the times, like we are on the verge of something very extraordinary. For those who believe His Word, today's scripture tells us that the Lord Jesus Christ will transform our lowly bodies so that they will be like His glorious body!

The Lord is showing us again in the Word that this transforming, changing, transfiguring to be in His image, should begin to take place <u>now</u>. If you go back several weeks and reread the days where we studied the scriptures about being the bride of Christ, you see that the Word urges us to prepare. How better to be prepared to be a bride without spot or blemish than to be transformed like His glorious body!

And, the type and shadow of this transformation is found in the Old Testament too. When the Lord brought Israel out of Egypt, they were all healed and very wealthy! And, He sustained them that way - not even their clothes wore out - for forty years on the way to the Promised Land. The account does *not* tell us that they were changed *when* they reached the Promised Land, but they were changed *on the way*!

Beloved, remember the Israelite children. Passing by the desert (or the dessert), preparing for the wedding, or being transformed, isn't always easy! But, hey! Should I care anymore if it is not easy? Here's what I say about that:

> "But that matters little. What matters most to me is to finish what God started: the job the Master Jesus gave me of letting everyone I meet know all about this incredibly extravagant generosity of God."
>
> (Acts 20:24, The Message)

THE PICTURE OF HEALTH®
DAILY POWER PLAN™
Day 65

Psalm 106:20 (NIV)

> They exchanged their Glory for an image of a bull, which eats grass.

Selah (pause and reflect)

Yesterday we talked of our being transformed into His image, into the glorious church. Today I want to continue to discuss the idea of your image, but in slightly different context. Throughout the Old and New Testaments you will find scriptures addressing one's image and "images." Our "Power Verse™" for today is one of those verses. In this Psalm, the children of God had repeatedly moved away from God to worship idols, which they had crafted for themselves. (I think it is interesting to note that they did so from the abundance that God provided for them. *Selah!*)

The Greek word for "image" as it is used in Genesis 1:26-27, is "tselem" {tseh'-lem}, meaning "in the likeness, a type or shadow of, embodiment, conception." We have studied some on how we were created in His image and how we are being transfigured into His likeness. This word, "tselem," carries the meaning of something that one "is" or that one was "created as."

Today I want to look at another word for "image" from the Greek word "pecel" {peh'-sel}. This is the word used in our text today. This word carries the meaning of a *graven* or engraved *object*, something that is *carved or hewn* from <u>natural material</u>. (Selah.) In contrast to "tselem," this word, "pecel," carries the meaning of something one has "formed" or "fashioned."

Beloved, the definitions of these two words are vitally important. You must discover in the Word what your true "image" is and *from that* determine what you should look and be like. You must also discover which "image" is driving your actions and choices because *its root will determine your results.*

Psalm 39:6 (YLT) says, "Only, in an image *{pecel}* doth each walk habitually, only, [in] vain, they are disquieted, He heapeth up and knoweth not who gathereth them." Beloved, that is the outcome for those who walk in the *mere, empty, semblance* of mental pictures *carved* into their minds, formed *by the ideals and idols of the world. Don't be fooled!* The enemy has carefully orchestrated the visual environment so that people will absorb deceptive "images." Our eyes have the opportunity hundreds of times each day to be exposed to these false representations designed to engrave a certain mental portrait of what is healthy, attractive, or desirable.

Think about it. How many Christians do we have today that are mentally and physically pursuing the "image" carved into their mind by the world? Or the images of success and beauty that were imprinted on young minds by someone else's remarks? Or the flawless, airbrushed images portrayed as real people by print advertising and media? Or even the image contained in the memory of one's own personal appearance or physical status in days gone by? Perhaps the image of what you looked like or weighed when you were in high school, the day you were married, or before you had children, etc?

Psalm 39:6 shows us that if we are pursuing these kinds of images, we are walking habitually in vain! That means we will never achieve that desired image. Deuteronomy 4:15-16 (NIV) clearly gives us the Lord's instruction:

> You saw no form of any kind the day the LORD spoke to you at Horeb out of the fire. Therefore *watch yourselves very carefully, so that you do not become corrupt and make for yourselves an idol, an image of any shape*, whether formed like a man or a woman…

Interesting. "Whether formed like a man or a woman…" What else is it, beloved, when we compare ourselves with others? It is carving into our hearts an image that is in complete conflict with His design and desire. Colossians 3:9 (NIV) says that when you are in Christ, you are to have "*taken off your old self with its practices and have put on the new self, which is being renewed in knowledge in the image* {"tselem"} *of its Creator.*"

Meditate on God's Word today. Find yourself *in* Him and let the Truth renew your mind *and* your heart regarding your *true* image ("tselem"). It is He who created us and not we who are crafting or forming ourselves! I encourage you to surrender your "idols" to Him. Let Him bring you revelation and, where needed, repentance. He is faithful to forgive and restore us if we will humble ourselves, turn from wicked, worldly ways, and worship Him alone!

THE PICTURE OF HEALTH®
DAILY POWER PLAN™

Day 66

2 Timothy 1:9 (NIV)

> "...who has saved us and called us to a holy life–not because of anything we have done but because of his own purpose and grace. This grace was given us in Christ Jesus before the beginning of time."

<u>*Selah (pause and reflect*</u>

Why is it that the very words "holy life" or "holiness" seem to bother so many people? Perhaps it is because they picture a legalistic, deprived life void of all fun or enjoyment. Or, perhaps others think it takes too much work to be holy. And still others think it is a lofty, unattainable goal, so why bother?

These views on holiness reveal the impact of man's false teaching about the subject. If you study holiness in the Bible, you will find that the true holiness is none of those things.

Easton's Bible dictionary says,

> "Holiness in the highest sense belongs to God (Isaiah 6:3; Rev 15:4), and to Christians as *consecrated to God's service*, and <u>**in so far as they are conformed in all things to the will of God**</u> (Rom 6:19,22; Eph 1:4; Tts 1:8; 1Pe 1:15). ***Personal holiness is a work of gradual development.*** It is carried on under many hindrances, hence the frequent

admonitions to watchfulness, prayer, and perseverance (1Cr 1:30; 2Cr 7:1; Eph 4:23,24)."

Holiness can be simply defined as "Christ-likeness", being like Christ. If we are "called to a holy life", to be like Christ, we must ask, "What then is Christ like?"

We know from scripture that Christ was *not religious*. In fact, the religious spirit of the Pharisees (pretense of holiness through appearances, words, and works) angered him. So what they displayed was not true holiness.

On the contrary, true holiness is the image of God seen in us, the power of the Spirit at work in us, and the gospel of Christ alive in us. It is *not* unattainable and the Lord has already done all the work!

We are made righteous through the Blood of Christ. Holiness can be looked at as the walking out of that righteousness by our everyday choices. Sometimes it is called the process of sanctification - a gradual development of holiness in your life as you *deliberately choose* to surrender more and more of your life to the will of God. But holiness - the display of His image in us - is only achieved in us as we willingly and faithfully obey His direction.

We don't have to work for it.

We do have to desire Him to change us and obey His instructions.

He desires to bring us up to a higher place in Him. Personal holiness is the way to that place. I encourage you to open your heart and yield yourselves to His instruction. Have the confidence in Him to see where He is longing to take us! As we do, we will see and experience life and health in measures beyond compare!

Truly, truly, glorious splendor awaits!

THE PICTURE OF HEALTH®
DAILY POWER PLAN™
Day 67

Jonah 2:7-9 (NIV)

> When my life was ebbing away, I remembered you, LORD, and my prayer rose to you, to your holy temple. Those who cling to worthless idols forfeit the grace that could be theirs. But I, with a song of thanksgiving, will sacrifice to you. What I have vowed I will make good. Salvation comes from the LORD.

Selah (pause and reflect

My excitement and passion, inspired by the Lord's handiwork, is the reason my heart brings this message to you today. So many people still stumble and remain in a defeated, mediocre life. Year after year is spent without victory, just lukewarm or worse, because they refuse to surrender the self-indulgent, rebellious attitude of the carnal nature to the authority of the Holy Spirit.

The classic example of this is related in the stories of at least three different friends and patients in the past year. Here is the general scenario: These people each have been telling me for the past year, or maybe two, that the Lord has been prompting them to healthier lifestyle habits. To one it is to increase vegetables; to another, it is to get off the junk food, stop the fast food, or get off the soda. I can't count how many times each of these people have come to the clinic and/or the classes and asked for advice on the same problems over and over. Each of them will start the process, but then every time they do, it's the same result...they failed to remain faithful to do what the Lord has instructed.

Now, I didn't say they failed. I said they failed to remain faithful, meaning they chose not to stay the course. (Remember Jonah, who ended up in the belly of the whale?) And, by the way, I forgot to tell you that all these friends and patients have each already once been made victors by the Lord's healing grace over previous cancers.

Typically, the next conversation goes something like this: "Oh Michelle, I am so sorry I dropped off the plan! I just can't seem to get on track. I am just too busy. I know the Lord knows where I am though and He understands." Sooner or later though, they will see the results of the mistaken assumption that it hasn't really cost them that much not to follow through.

See, many people have this mistaken attitude that God is amused or tolerant **_by reason of His grace_** of our rebelliousness, laziness, or careless abuse of the body, which is His dwelling place...created for His purpose. This is a lie, a deception, which we are going to set straight right now. Here is the truth from the Word of God:

The Lord *is* gracious and merciful. His love sent Christ to the cross to pay for your sins. The Lord Jesus suffered **every** temptation common to man. So, yes, *He does understand* like no one else what tempts us. ***But*** what He really understands is that *He has equipped you to overcome* them by His very own Blood and the power of the Spirit of God within you!

The Bible says in James 1:14-15, "...but each one is tempted when, by his own evil desire, he is dragged away and enticed. Then, after desire has conceived, it gives birth

to sin; and sin, when it is full grown, gives birth to death."
And then James 4:17 tells us plainly,

> *"Anyone, then, who knows the good he ought to do and doesn't do it, sins."*

My friends, we are *not* helpless to temptation of *any* kind! The Lord says in 2 Corinthians 12:9, *"My grace is sufficient for you, for my power is made perfect in weakness."* God's grace equips us to overcome temptation. His grace is <u>not</u> an excuse to knowingly and deliberately disobey God.

It is by no means humorous to Him when people who profess to love Him use His grace to justify blatant disobedience to the Father or to pretend to be helpless in overcoming temptation. In fact, the Word tells us exactly how He feels about it:

> *How much more severely do you think a man deserves to be punished who has trampled the Son of God under foot, who has treated as an unholy thing the blood of the covenant that sanctified him, and who has insulted the Spirit of grace?* (Hebrews 10:29 NIV)

Now, be careful that you don't misunderstand me; we are not speaking of someone who just makes a mistake. His mercy and grace allow that we are *being made* perfect, not yet having achieved it in full measure.

No, today's message is speaking to deliberate and repeated disobedience and rebellion. We must take it to heart that we have *an obligation to His grace not to live according to the sin nature but according to the Spirit who dwells in us.* (Romans 8:12)

Holiness is a work of gradual development, forward progress with a humble, willing heart. It is not some game of make-believe religion that mocks His grace.

How do you know the difference between a faithful effort and a rebellious choice? Romans 8:5 tells us:

> Those who live according to the sinful nature have their minds set on what that nature desires; but those who live in accordance with the Spirit have their minds set on what the Spirit desires.

Those who have their minds set on what the Spirit desires are equipped to overcome temptation. And, if you stumble (not deliberate disobedience) and your heart is set on God, there is conviction (not condemnation) that leads the humble heart to repentance. *That* is what qualifies for grace and mercy.

The truth is the things we place first in our lives are the things we honor and the things we worship. We will either worship God or idols, and perhaps it is time for some of you to admit that those idols are food and drink that are violating the temple. Jonah 2:8 from the passage above tells us, "Those who cling to worthless idols ***forfeit the grace*** that could be theirs."

This is a word of correction to many in the Body of Christ today. Will you receive it? Paul tells us in 2 Corinthians 5:17, "Therefore, if anyone is in Christ, he is a new creation; the old has gone, the new has come!" And then in 2 Corinthians 7:1 he urges us, "Since we have these promises, dear friends, let us purify ourselves from everything that contaminates body and spirit, perfecting holiness out of reverence for God."

Everyday I witness how the truth of His Word is actually restructuring my physical body. This same wonderful gift is available to every Believer. It is a provision that is ours to receive.

And what if you are one who has taken advantage of His grace? Earnestly repent and receive His forgiveness. His promise and provision are still there waiting for you. As you reach to Him with a willing heart, He will respond. As you walk in obedience to the Word, your life will be restored!

THE PICTURE OF HEALTH®
DAILY POWER PLAN™
Day 68

Ephesians 4:22-24 (AMP)

> Strip yourselves of your former nature [put off and discard your old un-renewed self] which characterized your previous manner of life and becomes corrupt through lusts and desires that spring from delusion;
>
> And be constantly renewed in the spirit of your mind [having a fresh mental and spiritual attitude],
>
> And put on the new nature (the regenerate self) created in God's image, [Godlike] in true righteousness and holiness.

Selah (pause and reflect

As yesterday's word of correction from the Lord pierced through the darkness in many hearts, it challenged me also to step up my own walk, to hold myself to a higher standard than before, to reach with a full heart toward God for increase, and to believe Him for measure that will honor His greatness.

Today as I write, I felt led to Ephesians 4:22-24. Again in my heart He ministers this message to lay down the desires and lusts that spring from delusion. But the Lord doesn't stop there. He wants us truly and completely free.

So many people have been deceived into thinking that the Christian walk is about what you give up or how you are deprived, especially when it comes to your health. That couldn't be farther from the truth! This lie goes so deep that people actually feel justified in pitying themselves for what they are doing without, like it is a badge of courage or something. What they don't see is how that mindset opens the door for the enemy to rob them in every area of their lives.

Christianity isn't about deprivation!

Beloved, He is teaching us the right ways in order to bring us up to greater victory and fulfillment! The Word is full of what He replaces in our lives when we put off the old self. His way of holiness brings us a fresh mental and spiritual attitude. (Who doesn't need that?!) He brings us hope for each day! He orders and directs our steps in wisdom.

Yes, this transformation into His image gives us a whole new nature to put on. It is like a new set of clothes. In truth, it is a new garment of skin, hair, nails, twinkling eyes, strong heart and lungs, healthy cells, gorgeous legs, and whatever you'd like in your new, regenerated body!

Beloved, what we are speaking of here is the restoration and resurrection of His perfect plan for your life, including your health! The shed Blood of Christ and His resurrection restore *all* that was given up in the Garden of Eden by man's sin...*all* of it.

He has given us the keys to His kingdom and invited us to partake of this glorious feast He has prepared for those who love Him and are called according to His purpose.

It is our choice whether or not to enter in and partake.

Don't be deluded any longer. Romans 8:26 says that the [Holy] Spirit comes to our aid and bears us up in our weakness. So, ask for His aid! Draw on His power today and strip off those old stinky rags! Lay down the "just get-by, take whatever disease comes my way, looking older every day" life and lay hold of the treasures in the Lord. Allow the power of God to change you and you will never desire nor ever miss those "worthless idols" again!

THE PICTURE OF HEALTH®
DAILY POWER PLAN™
Day 69

Ecclesiastes 7:10 (ESV)

> Say not, "Why were the former days better than these?" For it is not from wisdom that you ask this.

Selah (pause and reflect

Today was glorious! The weather was absolutely perfect! I spent the entire day working in the yard, trimming tall trees on a ladder, hauling the limbs away, raking leaves and bagging them - nine bags from just my flower bed, which has very few flowers and lots of leaves. What a transformation!

Sure the yard is making a little progress, but what I noticed the most change in was... me! It has been a long time since I had the desire to do anything like I did today and even longer since I had the strength and energy. And, here it is evening and I am not yet tired!

Amazing. Am I boasting? Yes I am, but *not* in me! This is so awesome because it has to be what the Lord is doing in me! There is just no other way I can be gaining the strength and stamina I felt today. So, yes, I boast in the Lord all day long! (Ps 44:8)

I share my awesome day with you to ask this, "Why would I ever look back and long for anything I laid down in order to get to this wonderful place?" Often as we make changes, we are tempted to say, "Oh, I wish I could have just one of those" or, "I'd love to have such and such", or, "wouldn't (any unhealthy habit) be good right now?" or even, "I miss having this or that." Our scripture today tells us that it is not wise to do so!

Beloved, we are being delivered out of the kingdom of darkness in to the kingdom of God's dear Son! (Colossians 1:13) We are daily being snatched away from the enemy's attempt to steal, kill, and destroy us. As we are, it is imperative that we recognize the changes and rejoice because of them. Giving thanks and praise to God for what He is doing in our bodies and our lives builds our faith. When we are continually giving praise to Him in front of others for each victory, we actually are guarding our hearts from turning back.

2 Peter 2:20 (NIV) tells us, "If they have escaped the corruption of the world by knowing our Lord and Savior Jesus Christ and are again entangled in it and overcome, they are worse off at the end than they were at the beginning." And then John, chapter 5, records the story of Jesus healing a man *who had suffered with affliction for 38 years.* John 5:14 (NIV) says, "...Jesus found him at the temple and said to him, 'See, you are well again. Stop sinning or something worse may happen to you.'"

Remember? We saw this very same thing in our text two days ago when three patients, all who had been previously healed of cancer, continued to make choices in direct disobedience to the Lord's instruction. Oh! Children of God! I plead with you to hear me and hear the Word of the Lord on this. It is the carnal, un-renewed nature that returns to sin - to idols which we worship instead of the Lord - again and again *even* when it knows the result will be great disease and destruction.

2 Corinthians 6:16 (NIV) asks us,

> What agreement is there between the temple of God and idols? For we are the temple of the living God. As God has said, "I will live with them and walk among them, and I will be their God, and they will be my people."

Isn't that a magnificent statement from Almighty God? Say it again. "I will live with them and walk among them, and I will be their God, and they will be my people."

You can build yourself up in this by putting that on your lips and in your ears, over and over. Thank Him for it out loud. Say, "Thank you, Lord. You, Almighty God, live with me and walk with me. Thank you that you are my God and I am your child, and my body is your dwelling place, the temple of your Holy Spirit. Transform me into your image, oh, God, with glorious splendor!"

Now, allow that truth to be made *real* in your heart and in your life today. Ask the Lord for it to be so. Let it penetrate to the very core of every cell and you will never be the same again. When it does, you will certainly not long for the wasteland of a life nor the body you left behind to walk with God!

THE PICTURE OF HEALTH®
DAILY POWER PLAN™

Day 70

Psalm 127:2 (AMP)

> It is vain for you to rise up early, to take rest late, to eat the bread of [anxious] toil—for He gives [blessings] to His beloved in sleep.

Selah (pause and reflect)

He gives His beloved blessed sleep. So why do so many suffer lack of sleep, sleeplessness, and sleep disorders? And beyond those, many more suffer diseases related to their lack of sleep than they realize. There are obvious sleep-related diseases like Chronic Fatigue and Sleep Apnea. But then there are not-so-obvious diseases connected to lack of sleep or poor sleep patterns such as depression, fibromyalgia, diabetes, menopausal difficulties and hormone imbalances, loss of sexual desire, hair loss, anxiety attacks, obesity...the list could go on and on!

What are we to do? As always, the Lord gives us the answers in His Word if we will only turn to it! For example, our verse for today gives us enormous insight into several root causes of sleep disturbances. Watch this!

First, the psalmist calls it *vanity* to lose sleep or allow things to rob us of proper sleep and rest! So, I looked up that word in the Greek and found it to mean emptiness, vanity, and/or falsehood. The expanded meaning is emptiness, nothingness, vanity, lying (deception), and worthlessness (of conduct). Wow! That certainly makes it plain.

Allowing anything or anyone to steal our peaceful sleep is worthless conduct.

Now, let's examine the next phrase from our scripture, "to eat the bread of sorrows". This phrase refers to something, an emotion or thought, which robs us of sleep. The meaning of this in the Greek indicates it is a hurt, pain, toil, sorrow, labor, hardship, offense, or - get this - *an idol*! (Didn't we just study about *worthless idols*?)

So the Word shows us that it is worthless conduct and even lying to ourselves when we allow hurts, pain, offense, or idols to rob us of sleep. It is worthless because it is not of faith, love, or forgiveness. It is worthless because it steals our health and peace.

But *the Lord!* The Lord gives us "blessed" and "sweet" sleep! If we are choosing anything else, we are rejecting knowledge and His wise provision! (We studied the results from that previously as well!)

In our fast paced, 24-7 world, I believe the Lord is beckoning us to return to claim our glorious inheritance - His provision, His blessings, His gifts. As we study the scriptures this week about rest and sleep, incline your ear to hear Him calling,

"Come unto me all ye that labour and are heavy laden, and I will give you rest."

(Mathew 11:28KJV)

THE PICTURE OF HEALTH®
DAILY POWER PLAN™
Day 71

Isaiah 14:3 (KJV)

> And it shall come to pass in the day that the LORD shall give thee rest from thy sorrow, and from thy fear, and from the hard bondage wherein thou wast made to serve...

Selah (pause and reflect)

Did you know that "insufficiency" is one of the three primary causes of disease and dysfunction? It is true. All disease and dysfunction of the body can be traced back to its root in at least one of three general categories: insufficiency, toxicity, and trauma.

There are seven certain essentials that are required by the body in order to produce health. Sleep is one of the body's seven essential requirements. When you sleep, it is the set time for your body to rest, repair, and rebuild.

For example, certain organs like liver and gallbladder do their cleansing and maintenance nightly between the hours of 11:00pm and 2:00am. Muscles rest and clear themselves of lactic acid from the day's activities. Certain hormones that impact your moods are produced during this time. Growth hormone, anti-aging activities, and thyroid function are impacted by sleep patterns as well.

The key, however, is that these functions occur optimally only when you are *asleep*. So, what if you do not sleep or do not sleep with sufficient quantity and quality? You open the door for disease and dysfunction to begin.

We began studying yesterday that vanity, worthless conduct, sorrows and pain, offense, and hurt all rob us of sleep. We find this repeated in Ecclesiastes 2:23,

> **For all his days are sorrows, and his travail grief; yea, his heart taketh not rest in the night. This is also vanity.**

Beloved, the enemy has quietly robbed health from God's people for years in the area of rest and sleep because of their own vanity. Well, I say, "Not any more!" In bringing us to these scriptures, the Lord is exposing this attempt to destroy us and He is leading us to the Word that makes us free.

The Word of God from Isaiah says *the Lord shall give* us **rest** *from* sorrow, from fear, and from hard bondage. He shall give it. He desires to set you free from that bondage. Will you let him? In Matthew 11:29(KJV), He even tells us, "Take my yoke upon you, and learn of me; for I am meek and lowly in heart: and ye shall find rest unto your souls."

In a world of people who are sick and tired, this day we can take His yoke and learn of Him and find that rest. As we do, beloved, we will awake and behold that He has replenished and refreshed the weary! We will find our sleep is sweet. (Jeremiah 31:26)

The Picture of Health® Daily Power Plan™

Day 72

Psalm 16:9 (AMP)

> Therefore my heart is glad and my glory
> [my inner self] rejoices; my body too shall
> rest and confidently dwell in safety…

Selah (pause and reflect)

Did you notice that this is another example of the "connection", the communion of our Spirit, Soul, and Body that we learned about several weeks ago? Over and over you will see how the blessings of God flow from one area to the others and back again.

This beautiful scripture brings out that His provision reaches our heart, which is the soul, but also the inner self (the spirit) *and* the body. The Psalmist says "my body too" rests and confidently dwells in safety!

Beloved, it is rest in your soul that allows your body to rest and sleep sweetly. Rest in your soul refreshes your spirit. This principle also works in the negative. The psalmist tells us in Psalm 38:3, "There is no soundness in my flesh because of Your indignation; neither is there any health or rest in my bones because of my sin."

When God created the heavens and the earth, He set forth the pattern for us in work, play, and rest. He chose, as recorded in Genesis 1, to set an example by spreading out the "labor" over six days and on the seventh day He rested. There were breaks between workdays, there was pleasure and enjoyment as He looked upon His work, was pleased, and said it was good. And, there was rest from labor.

I know in my life this is an area He is growing me and teaching me of its purpose and its value, and, I am glad. I can testify that it is setting me free from years of bondage that left my body and my emotions exhausted and my heart resentful. But no more! I am learning to rest in Him, to play more, and, yes, to work.

One thing that has helped me greatly in correcting my work perspective comes from Ephesians 4:28. Instead of following my own way, I am learning to rest and to work in the fruitful labor of love that His path provides for me. Instead of working to make a living, the right heart toward God works to give and sows to live!

As we continue to study the Word on rest and sleep, give some thought to *your* days. Do you have balance between work, play, and rest? Does your sleep allow the body to heal and be refreshed? Leave out the excuses and the justifications and ask the Lord what *He says* about that area of your life. As He shows you the changes to make and you respond, you can be confident that His presence will be with you. As you seek Him, He will cause you to triumph and He will bring you blessed sleep!

THE PICTURE OF HEALTH®
DAILY POWER PLAN™
Day 73

Exodus 20:11 (NIV)

> For in six days the LORD made the heavens and the earth, the sea, and all that is in them, but he rested on the seventh day. Therefore the LORD blessed the Sabbath day and made it holy.

<u>Selah (pause and reflect)</u>

Years ago, I owned a consulting business. It was my practice to spend one or two nights a month working all night at the office. I reasoned that, because I was a "night person", I was much more productive during those nights and I could make up the lost sleep on the weekends. Without employees and the telephone interrupting me every few minutes I could plow through piles of work in those quiet hours!

What I didn't know is that there is truly no such thing as a "night person". The whole design of our maintenance system was purposefully linked, by The Creator, to the circadian rhythm, the day and night cycle of the earth, the sun, and the moon or night.

My actions or habits were in direct conflict with God's design of my body and desire for my life. I had no concept of the toll my lifestyle was taking on my health but it wasn't long before the result of this conflict began to show. Every late night's work prevented precious healing from happening in my body and symptoms began to appear.

Although I was young and still not showing the aging effects, other areas of my health were suffering. My emotions became more easily provoked and less stable. My body ached with the pains of fibromyalgia and chronic fatigue. I had forgotten how to laugh and enjoy life. Though I didn't smoke and rarely had alcohol, I existed on adrenaline, sugar, and caffeine. I was the classic case of burning my candle at both ends!

Eventually, that candle began to burn in two and I desperately cried out to the Lord for help. As I studied the Word, I found that God in His design of the earth and man set forth the precedent of rest. Even the Almighty God did not create everything on the first day, but divided up the work and rest periods, separating day from night. He wrote it down for us in Genesis 1:14, "And God said, 'Let there be lights in the expanse of the sky to separate the day from the night, and let them serve as signs to mark seasons and days and years,'".

The Lord set forth the pattern for us when He ceased from His labor with a final long rest on the seventh day. It really shouldn't amaze us then that following this pattern with our physical bodies helps to produce optimal health. God blessed this day of rest and made it holy. That alone should speak to us that this is important, a pattern to which we should give our attention! Repeated rebellion toward the body's God-given design (in harmony with the earth's circadian rhythms) is sin and will produce disease, premature destruction, and eventually, death.

The Lord in His grace and mercy has taught me about the importance of sleep. Placing Him first and making rest and sleep a priority has restored to me a life of peace, joy, and health. I can truly say that, although I am now twelve years older than the days described above, I look and feel younger than I have in years.

If you are having difficulty sleeping, unable to fall asleep, wake up too often, or don't feel well-rested when you wake up in the morning, consider that a "wake-up" call from your body that something is not right! Don't just ignore the indicators of disease or accept them as "just how I am", "how I've always been", or "something I have to tolerate."

"Return unto thy rest, O my soul; for the LORD hath dealt bountifully with thee."

Psalm 116:7 (KJV)

In His love, He is making us aware of this essential requirement for health. We have a great commission to attend to. We must have proper sleep and rest to fulfill the purpose to which we are called. Take heed today of the Lord's command that there be rest in your life. Determine today to study the scriptures on sleep and rest so that His desire and purpose may be more fully manifested in your life.

THE PICTURE OF HEALTH®
DAILY POWER PLAN™

Day 74

Selah (pause and reflect)

I came upon this Psalm while studying the scriptures on The Breath of Life, to breathe, and breathing. This translation of Psalm 34 in the Message Bible is extraordinary and struck me deeply as exactly what we needed to hear today.

The passage note tells us this is a psalm of David, a poem called an acrostic where each verse begins with consecutive letters of the Hebrew alphabet. But the really important note is that this is a psalm of praise and victory because David had escaped the clutches of bondage and death! (Yes, exactly what we have escaped! Praise the Lord!)

I urge you to read these verses out loud, to make it personal as you speak it back to God with the emotion of your heart, and to let the Lord speak to you today in these many powerful statements of praise and victory! (Emphasis added.)

Psalm 34 (The Message)

I bless GOD every chance I get; my lungs expand with his praise.

I live and breathe GOD;

if things aren't going well, hear this and be happy:

Join me in spreading the news; together let's get the word out.

GOD met me more than halfway; he freed me from my anxious fears.

Look at him; give him your warmest smile. Never hide your feelings from him.

When I was desperate, I called out, and GOD got me out of a tight spot.

GOD's angel sets up a circle of protection around us while we pray.

Open your mouth and taste, open your eyes and see—how good GOD is.

Blessed are you who run to him.

Worship GOD if you want the best; worship opens doors to all his goodness.

Young lions on the prowl get hungry, but GOD-seekers are full of God.

Come, children, listen closely; I'll give you a lesson in GOD worship.

Who out there has a lust for life? Can't wait each day to come upon beauty?

Guard your tongue from profanity, and no more lying through your teeth.

Turn your back on sin; do something good. Embrace peace—don't let it get away!

GOD keeps an eye on his friends; his ears pick up every moan and groan.

GOD won't put up with rebels; he'll cull them from the pack.

Is anyone crying for help?

GOD is listening, ready to rescue you.

If your heart is broken, you'll find GOD right there;

if you're kicked in the gut, he'll help you catch your breath.

Disciples so often get into trouble; still, GOD is there every time.

He's your bodyguard, shielding every bone; not even a finger gets broken.

The wicked commit slow suicide; they waste their lives hating the good.

GOD pays for each slave's freedom;

No one who runs to him loses out.

THE PICTURE OF HEALTH®
DAILY POWER PLAN™
Day 75

Job 33:4 (KJV)

> The spirit of God hath made me, and the breath of the Almighty hath given me life.

Selah (pause and reflect)

Hallelujah! The breath of the Almighty has given me life! (Indeed, He has!)

While studying on the body's essential requirement of breath, I found that the Bible refers to the Breath of God, the Breath of Life, and the Breath of the Almighty repeatedly. I learned that He uses his breath to inspire, as is recorded in 2 Timothy 3:16 (KJV), "All scripture is given by inspiration (breath) of God, and is profitable for doctrine, for reproof, for correction, for instruction in righteousness." Other verses teach us that His breath is used to destroy the wicked (Job 4:8-10). And many verses show us that His breath was used to create the heavens and the earth (Psalm 33:6, Psalm 18:15, Gen 1:6, Ps 148:5, Heb 11:3).

I was intrigued by these many examples of how God's breath is powerful to give life or to destroy. I thought, if we then recall that we are made in His image, we can better comprehend that our breath contains this same power to give our physical bodies life or, in the absence of breath, death!

Your breathing acquires and transports oxygen, which is the fuel every cell needs for life. Just like your first breath, each new breath continues the process through which we produce energy to heal, to remove toxins, and to transport nutrients that support the healthy function of our entire body. With full, deep, quality breaths, we live and flourish in health. Without them, we die.

The Bible tells us in Romans 8:11 (KJV) that "if the Spirit of him that raised up Jesus from the dead dwell in you, he that raised up Christ from the dead shall also quicken your mortal bodies by his Spirit that dwelleth in you." And the Bible also tells us in 1Corinthians 6:14 that the power, the Breath of Life, which raised Christ from the dead, will also raise us up!

As we study about breathing and its importance to our health, let us be guided and impressed by God's example. Through His Word and His Holy Spirit, He is teaching us about the function of breath in our physical bodies, to take His instruction and, literally, breathe new life into our mortal bodies!

THE PICTURE OF HEALTH®
DAILY POWER PLAN™
Day 76

Ezekiel 37:4-6 (NLT)

> Then he said to me, "Speak to these bones and say, 'Dry bones, listen to the word of the LORD! This is what the Sovereign LORD says: Look! I am going to breathe into you and make you live again! I will put flesh and muscles on you and cover you with skin. I will put breath into you, and you will come to life. Then you will know that I am the LORD.'"

Selah (pause and reflect)

Our first act when we emerge from the womb is to inspire. Our last act is to dis-inspire or expire. These breaths, first in and finally out, are like parentheses that encompass our physical life. It should be no surprise then that breath would be so remarkably linked to *the power of healing*.

This breath, the very thing that supplies my daily life, comes from Him and is part of His excellent design of the wondrous human body. Did you know it is breath that moves the River of Life in your body, the spinal fluids that course from the top of your head to the tip of your tailbone? Yes, the breathing action is actually the pump that causes the current of that river to move up and down the spinal column, supplying life to the whole body. Not only that, but it regulates the beat of your heart and the pumping of blood, which also gives life to your body.

Can you hear the Lord speaking to you about this today? Beloved, He desires above all things that you prosper and be in health! Today, He is reaching out to you with this message. He desires to give new life to your body. For it is written, "This is what the Sovereign LORD says: 'Look! I am going to breathe into you and make you live again! I will put flesh and muscles on you and cover you with skin. I will put breath into you, and you will come to life. Then you will know that I am the LORD.'"

Receive that word from Him today, beloved. It was meant for you.

The Lord told the prophet in Ezekiel 37:9 to speak it (out loud) as a command. As he did, the dead bodies, dry bones, were made alive again. In the same way, you and I should also declare it to be so! Start now! Speak it boldly to your body, and, for that matter, to everyone who is around you, proclaim new life into you to His glory:

> "Thank you, Lord! You are breathing life into me and making me live again! Thank you that You are giving me healthy bones, strong muscles, and covering me with beautiful, healthy skin! I speak that my body is receiving and walking in fullness of life in every area so that I, and all who see me, will know that You are the Lord! Glory be to God, who heals me and gives me life!"

THE PICTURE OF HEALTH®
DAILY POWER PLAN™

Day 77

2 Corinthians 2:14-15 (The Message)

> And I got it, thank God! In the Messiah, in Christ, God leads us from place to place in one perpetual victory parade. Through us, he brings knowledge of Christ. Everywhere we go, people breathe in the exquisite fragrance. Because of Christ, we give off a sweet scent rising to God, which is recognized by those on the way of salvation—an aroma redolent with life.

Selah (pause and reflect

Ever walked past a bakery and smelled the wonderful aroma of fresh baked bread? We have a restaurant and bakery in my hometown called *Neighbor's Mill*™. They bake from scratch the most delicious and healthy bread you can put in your mouth! At least one morning each week my husband and I stop by for breakfast just after they have baked the day's fresh bread. And Oh! What a fragrance! Smells so good you just have to taste it!

That is how our lives should be to those around us! We should be such a sweet aroma of the love of God that others are drawn to breathe it in! Our verse today says we are a sweet scent rising to God, as are our prayers (Rev. 5:8). Elsewhere the scriptures also tell us, "To those who are perishing we are a fearful smell of death and doom. But to those who are being saved we are a life-giving perfume..." (2 Cor 2:16 NLT)

What does that have to do with your health? You see, beloved, it is *His victory revealed in our lives* that produces the aroma "redolent with life", the life-giving, exquisite fragrance of the knowledge of Christ.

When we walk in the light of revelation the Lord has given us, our spirit, soul, and body prosper. To other people, that prosperity, that magnificent health, is *a visible sign of the love of God, the redemption through Christ, and the power of the Holy Spirit.* It *beckons* them to breathe it in and ask you, "What is that exquisite aroma in your life?"

My friend, when that happens, your health just became your witness for Christ.

Child of God, *now* is the time for us to be His witnesses, *not just in word*, but also in deed. We are, after all, His ambassadors to the world (2 Corinthians 5:20). Now is the time for us to lay hold of the victory He purchased and *for our lives to be proof of His power that worketh in us*!

I appeal to you today to completely yield your life to Him and watch His power bring it to pass! If you are willing and obedient, He will surely lead you from place to place in one perpetual victory parade. Rise up and allow the love of God, the light of Christ, and the power of the Holy Spirit to manifest as radiant health in your physical body. Every step, every choice, every day, activate the revelation of the Word of God to give you confidence to stand firm in your walk, making the choices that produce health in your body *so that* He is glorified!

THE PICTURE OF HEALTH® DAILY POWER PLAN™
Day 78

1 Corinthians 2:14 (AMP)

> But the natural, nonspiritual man does not accept or welcome or admit into his heart the gifts and teachings and revelations of the Spirit of God, for they are folly (meaningless nonsense) to him; and he is incapable of knowing them [of progressively recognizing, understanding, and becoming better acquainted with them] because they are spiritually discerned and estimated and appreciated.

Selah (pause and reflect)

Every once and a while, I will have a conversation with someone about health or about *The Picture of Health*® programs and I come away thinking, "Lord, they just don't get it! Why is this not reaching them?" I feel like I have just spoken Japanese to them and it went in one ear and out the other.

Usually it is a "dieter" who just wants to lose weight; therefore, they hear nothing I say about health. So, I mostly let those people go without too much effort. But then, there is the second group. The person in this group is someone who is a Christian, loves the Lord, reads the Word, maybe is even called and serving in ministry, and yet completely fails to see the importance of, and obligation to, attending to the care of their body as the temple of God. These really grieve my spirit! I think to myself, "Just how do they think they are going to 'go into all the world and reach the lost with the gospel of Christ' in a vessel that can't get across the room without pain or getting winded?" At the very least, their body doesn't exactly scream "Victory!" to those around them. What kind of witness is their physical body to the power of God?

Then I smile and remember that is the same question I heard in my own heart when I started this journey. And the Lord reminds me of this verse in 1 Corinthians 2:14. My favorite version of this verse is the Amplified (above). But I also like the Message, which reads, "The unspiritual self, just as it is by nature, can't receive the gifts of God's Spirit. There's no capacity for them. They seem like so much silliness. Spirit can be known only by spirit—God's Spirit and our spirits in open communion."

Before long, we will be nearing the completion of another 100-day session of *The Picture of Health*® program. The completion brings many emotions as I greet new friends just starting the journey and say goodbye to beloved brothers and sisters in Christ who are ready to go forth, now in glorious, restored health, to fulfill His purpose in their lives.

There are always some who stay on to bridge the gap between those groups, making their way through for the second, third, or even the eighth time, to continue building their faith and increasing in the understanding of His mighty power at work in their lives. And, yes, there are some that move on without ever understanding the purpose at all.

Whatever the case, by faith, I trust that, whether I ever personally see it or not, the seed planted will be watered by the Lord of the Harvest and the Word spoken in their lives will not return void but will accomplish that for which it was sent. Amen?

As we conclude this session, our final topics will be covering the last few of the seven essentials required for physical health, including "What You Think" and "What You Say". Like all the days before, your grasp or understanding of these lessons will depend on whether or not you choose to receive the loving gifts and direction from God's Spirit.

I share with you again, beloved, that it is about the pattern, the connection, and the communion. And, it is about your choices.

Your homework for today is to decide whether you will accept, welcome, or admit into your heart the gifts and teachings and revelations of the Spirit of God. Or, will you treat them as they are folly, meaningless nonsense? Will you consider His instruction and revelation as unimportant, silliness, or not applicable to you? Or, will you yield yourself to Him so that you progressively recognize, understand, and become better acquainted with God will and purpose for your life?

Now is the time of His approaching. There is a purpose and a commission to be fulfilled. Who will go forth for Him and prepare the way? Or perhaps I should ask it this way, *"Who will be able to?"*

And **I** said, "**Here** am **I. Send me!**" (Isaiah 6:8)

THE PICTURE OF HEALTH®
DAILY POWER PLAN™
Day 79

Colossians 1:28-29 (NIV)

> We proclaim him, admonishing and teaching everyone with all wisdom, so that we may present everyone perfect in Christ. To this end I labor, struggling with all his energy, which so powerfully works in me.

Selah (pause and reflect)

I was talking with a prayer partner of mine today who asked about the current projects I am working on with the Lord and I told her it was like being nine months pregnant (and counting) with your first child, so ready to deliver and excitedly trusting God to take you through! And it is. Like in our scripture for today, I am in labor for all of you, struggling with all His energy, to deliver this message, His wellness revelation for the end-time Body of Christ.

For several years now, I have understood that it is our calling through *The Picture of Health®* to proclaim, to admonish, and to teach in His wisdom *the complete liberty and healing* that is ours through Christ for the physical body, as well as for the spirit and soul. In that, I saw only in part. Now, by His grace and revelation, I see more fully and will share it with you over the next few days.

Do you remember how I have been sharing with you about the awesome changes happening in my body and in many of your bodies as well? And remember also that just two weeks ago (when we studied in Jonah) we read, "The *working* of holiness *in our lives transforms us*, and our physical body, into glorious splendor"?

Well, beloved, there is a measure of power we have been experiencing for weeks, you and I, as we've studied together, and I now have the description I have been searching for, to put words to this experience. I heard it in a dynamic message from a man of God just this last weekend and when I did, I knew immediately that it was and is that which is happening in our bodies as we seek Him... "It worketh in me!"

But first, there is something we need to address. I felt in my spirit this morning that some of you have wandered in your thinking, letting yourselves slip into "church" mode, or religious thinking, about these Daily Power Plans™. I encourage you to check yourselves, judge yourself, and make an attitude correction, if necessary, so you don't miss a thing! We are so instructed in 1 Corinthians 11:30-32 (NIV):

> "That is why many among you are weak and sick, and a number of you have fallen asleep. But if we judged ourselves, we would not come under judgment. When we are judged by the Lord, we are being disciplined so that we will not be condemned with the world."

This tool, called *The Picture of Health®*, which carries the Gospel, is about healing, liberty, and restoration. It is about the power that worketh in you, and in me, and how that literally *changes* your physical body. To lose sight of this truth is to miss the point of the revelation God is bringing us and *why* He is doing so. Each day as we study together, we should purpose to remember that we are endeavoring to learn His Word about our bodies *so that* we can possess the victory He desires and our commission requires.

Look at each scripture in light of what it means and brings to your physical health, in addition to your spirit and soul. As you do, you will begin to see the healing, resurrection power of God manifest in your physical body in greater measure than we've ever seen or even imagined! How will you know when it starts? How will you know if you are in faith about this and have the right heart to receive? You'll be excited!

Pray about that today and we'll take a deeper look at the power that 'worketh in us' when we study again tomorrow. Until then, stir yourself up in faith to eagerly desire His best for you and your body!

For homework, open your Bible to Isaiah 58 and read it out loud. As you read, look beyond the written words to their meaning, His intent, drinking in the message of what His Word is speaking in that chapter.

Don't forget! It isn't very long, so you should each take time to do it. Come tomorrow prepared to step up to a new measure of His power at work in you!

THE PICTURE OF HEALTH®
DAILY POWER PLAN™
Day 80

Isaiah 9:2 (NIV)

> The people walking in darkness have seen a great light; on those living in the land of the shadow of death (*or*, land of darkness) a light has dawned.

Selah (pause and reflect)

There are many of you right on the threshold of major breakthroughs. I believe, like our scripture for today says, "a light has dawned", and revelation has come. I believe that the power of that light has snatched you from darkness, the land of the shadow of death, and is renewing your mind and transforming your body, day by day.

Psalm 119:105 says, "Your word is a lamp to my feet and a light for my path." Psalm 119:130 tells us that "the unfolding of your words gives light; it gives understanding to the simple." I thank the Lord that His unfolding Word is giving us light and understanding, bringing us all into a greater measure of faith and health. Isaiah 2:5 beckons us,

"Come...let us walk in the light of the Lord!"

Yesterday, I introduced to you the description 'it worketh in me'. Let's believe together for the unfolding of His Word as we study that which 'worketh in us', where it comes from, and where it now abides. We're going to take it line upon line, precept upon precept, so that each of us can understand. It is my prayer that each of you will come to know the mystery of our glorious inheritance in Christ.

To start, Psalm 36:9 tells us that in God is the fountain of life and in His light we see light. 1John 1:5-7 tells us that "... God is light; in him there is no darkness at all. If we claim to have fellowship with him yet walk in the darkness, we lie and do not live by the truth. But if we walk in the light, as he is in the light, we have fellowship with one another, and the blood of Jesus, his Son, purifies us from all sin."

So God dwells in light, He is light, and in Him there is no darkness at all. Jesus told us in John 8:12, "I am the light of the world. Whoever follows me will never walk in darkness, but will have the light of life."

1Peter 2:9 goes further in saying that He "called you out of darkness into His wonderful light." Jesus *also* said in Matthew 5:14 that "**you** are the light of the world...." And, Ephesians 5:8 repeats that for us, "For you were once darkness, but now you *are light* in the Lord. Live as children of light." (Emphasis added.)

How does that connect with your physical health? I am going to bring us to that, but first you must better comprehend this word "light".

When you flip the light switch on at your house, what makes the light shine? Power. Without power, there is no light, correct? The light is actually energy, power, which is channeled through a vessel into a source of output. Energy particles translate into real, scientifically measurable *power*. In addition, science tells us that energy cannot be created (by man) only *transferred*. Remember this for later because this truth will be very important as we continue!

The scriptures establish that God *is* light - He doesn't just have light, but *He is light* - the source of all power in creation. All that was made was made by His power, the Light, through the Word (Gen 1:3, John 1:1). The Word also tells us that God *is* love (1 John 4:8). His perfect love is the ultimate energy source, the power, which is manifest in the person of Christ who is the light of the world and which is expressed through the person and power of the Holy Spirit (Acts 1:8).

By Christ's death, burial, and resurrection (accomplished through the power and love of God), the veil between God and man was torn in two, which made His power, His light, His love, and His Word available to all who will receive the magnificent gift of Christ as Savior. When we repent and accept that free gift of salvation, being baptized in the Name of Jesus Christ for the forgiveness of our sins, Acts 2:38 tells us that we receive the Holy Spirit. In Acts 1:8 it is written, "*You will receive power when the Holy Spirit comes upon you.*"

Look at this: When the angel of the Lord came to visit Mary, the mother of Jesus, he told her (Luke 1:35 NIV), "... The Holy Spirit will come upon you, and the power of the Most High will overshadow you." Mary invited the will of the Lord in her life by saying, "...may it be to me as you have said", and Mary became with child and gave birth to Jesus, who is the light of the world.

When you, by your invitation to Christ to be your Lord and Savior, become a born-again, child of God, the Holy Spirit comes upon *you* and there is again a new birth. However, unlike Mary's natural birthing of Jesus, this new birth takes place *in you* (Galatians 2:20), as you are made a new creation in Christ. At that moment of rebirth, you receive the Holy Spirit and become the light of the world as the body of Christ. Instead of a body being birthed *from* you, like Mary, His power was birthed *in you and you became His Body and His Light* (1Cor. 12:27, Mat 5:14, Romans 12:5, 1Cor.10:16, 1Cor.12:12).

This is that which *worketh in you.* Oh, friends, this is so powerful and so big! My heart longs to lay it all out for you today, but I can't. I do believe that the foundational truths we have laid thus far provide an excellent place to stop and meditate. I encourage you to look up the scriptures for yourself. As you meditate on what we have covered so far, let it penetrate your spirit, soul, and body with *fresh revelation* on **Christ in you: His light, His power, His Spirit.**

Stay with me and I know the Lord will bring us into fullness of revelation of this powerful truth!

THE PICTURE OF HEALTH®
DAILY POWER PLAN™
Day 81

Ephesians 3:20 (NIV)

> "Now to him who is able to do immeasurably more than all we ask or imagine, according to his power that is at work within us…"

Selah (pause and reflect)

Ever wish you could do something with your physical body? Live free from all sickness and disease? Overcome cancer? Lose or gain weight? Look younger and feel better? Repair the damage from years of abuse? Live to be one hundred twenty so that you can run the race, fulfill your full purpose, and finish strong? (That's my current favorite.)

We have established from the Word that God is light and power (and in Him, that is infinite power). We have also established in the Word that His light (which is power) is *in* the born-again child of God. Our scripture today tells us plainly that He is able to do **immeasurably more than all we ask or imagine,** *according to his power that is at work within us*!

If you have been studying daily with me, I know you have got to be getting excited, because you surely are beginning to see where this is going! (Yes, *this* is the place to shout!)

Beloved, this is what we call, "*Your Health: The Mystery Revealed!*" ™ It is the title of a companion book we've written for *The Picture of Health*®, but most importantly, it is your inheritance in Christ when He lives in you. You have the power abiding in you that is able to do more than all you can ask or imagine!

That is how Jesus could say in John 14:12, "I tell you the truth, anyone who has faith in me will do what I have been doing. He will do even greater things than these, because I am going to the Father." Jesus knew that when He went to the Father, the Holy Spirit was coming to dwell in us in power! He even told His disciples not to leave Jerusalem until the Holy Spirit came to them and they received that power (Acts 1:4).

Why is this a big deal for us? Because it is this power that worketh in us that will *cause* the victory to be *manifest* in our body! If you are a child of God, the power of God - the anointing - is already resident in you to do the work. 1 Thessalonians 2:13 says the Word of God is *at work in them who believe.* And, in Philippians 2:13 it is written, "... for it is God who *works in you* <u>to will and to act</u> **according to his good purpose**." (Emphasis added.)

When you comprehend that it is *real* and that He has transferred (made available in us) His power into us through the Holy Spirit, you will finally believe, and thus receive, the magnificent result.

Why is it so important that we get this and it be revealed (manifest) in our physical bodies? Because, beloved, I believe with all my heart, He is opening our eyes to His Word in this great day of His approaching *so that* we are made witnesses to all the world of His wondrous love and great power at work in our lives, in our bodies, in a measure which the world has never seen before and the likes of which we have never imagined!

Acts 17:28 says, "For *in him* we *live* and *move* and *have our being*". Never before was this so personally true and I sense that we have only just begun to comprehend it!

THE PICTURE OF HEALTH®
DAILY POWER PLAN™
Day 82

John 1:5 (KJV)

> And the light shineth in darkness; and the darkness comprehended it not.

Selah (pause and reflect)

The last few weeks, as we've been studying the power that worketh in us to will and to act according to His good purpose (Philippians 2:13), I have to think that at least one of you has wondered (again), "If this is true, why, then, are so many Christians still sick?" After all, doesn't John 8:12 say, "Then spake Jesus again unto them, saying, I am the light of the world: he that followeth me shall not walk in darkness, but shall have the *light of life*"? (Emphasis added.) The answer is found in John 1:5:

> **"…the light shineth in darkness; and the darkness *comprehended it not*".**

One's first thought might be to interpret the scripture above as they simply did not understand. However, according to Strong's concordance, the word "comprehend" is translated from the Greek word "katalambano" {kat-al-am-ban'-o}. It actually means, "to lay hold of, so as to make one's own, to obtain, attain to, *to take into one's self*, or to appropriate."

It also means to "seize upon, take possession of, as in: evils overtaking one, of the last day overtaking the wicked with destruction, of a demon about to torment one, or, in a good sense, of Christ by his holy power and influence laying hold of the human mind and will, in order to prompt and govern it, to detect, catch, and to lay hold of with the mind"[1]

This makes it clear that some remain in sickness or disease because they have not laid hold of, have not *made their own* or they *have not seized* the light (the power and knowledge) which is the healing power of God available in Christ through the Holy Spirit.

Do you remember when we studied the verse from Hosea 4:6, "...my people are destroyed from **lack** of knowledge"? We learned then that their lack of knowledge was actually because they had "rejected knowledge".

Why would anyone deliberately do that? John 3:19 (NIV) answers, "This is the verdict: Light has come into the world, but men *loved darkness instead of light* because their deeds were evil."

That is the key: *Comprehension* (revelation) about the power that worketh in you, and even the question as to whether it does work in you or not, *depends on what it is that you love.*

God is love. And He has freely offered His Son, Jesus Christ, the light, to you **so that** no one who believes in Him should stay in darkness (John 12:46). It is *love* - the source of His Glory, the light that is power - which activates your faith. It is written in Galatians 5:6 that **faith *worketh* by love**.

The bottom line is...*whatever you love most motivates your actions and your will.* In John 14:15 (NIV), Jesus said, "If you love me, you will obey what I command." If the power of God does *not* 'worketh' in you to the degree beyond all that you can ask or imagine, if it isn't yet a witness for the world to see that testifies to His Glory, perhaps there are things that you have loved more than Him.

I know that can be a touchy subject, but, lovingly I ask you, "Do you want to be free or not?" I believe you truly do. So, as we close for today, I ask you to examine your heart. Ask the Lord to reveal to you any area where you do not obey His commands, where you love anything else more than Him. As He shows you, repent and let Him turn you from darkness to light, and from the power of satan to God (Acts 26:18).

2 Chronicles 7:14 (KJV) tells us, "If my people, which are called by my name, shall humble themselves, and pray, and seek my face, and turn from their wicked ways; then will I hear from heaven, and will forgive their sin, and will heal their land." And 1 John 1:9 assures us that, "…if we confess our sins, he is faithful and just to forgive us our sins, and to cleanse us from all unrighteousness".

Beloved, "His divine power has given us everything we need for life and godliness through our knowledge of him who called us by his own glory and goodness" (2Peter 1:3 NIV). Jesus came that we might have life and have it more abundantly. Let us return His love, having no other gods before Him. Let us earnestly endeavor to walk in the light He has so freely given us, laying hold of, *comprehending*, *Christ in us*.

[1] KJV of Strong's Concordance #2638

THE PICTURE OF HEALTH®
DAILY POWER PLAN™

Day 83

Romans 8:28 (KJV)

> And we know that all things work together for good to them that love God, to them who are the called according to his purpose.

Selah (pause and reflect)

Yesterday, I was excitedly sharing with my husband about more of the changes taking place in my physical body and also the continuing revelation on the power that "worketh in me". I was trying to describe how the changes are not only physical, but that they are coming about because my mind, my soul, is being internally renewed with this revelation of God's truth to the degree that my actions and my will are being changed.

I was struggling, as I am now, to accurately describe the amazing transformation I am witnessing. I was trying to put into words the process that is causing it to happen. See, the power of God is working in my physical body to change it, but the power is also working in my mind to cause my choices, my actions, to be for His purpose and good pleasure.

So, it worketh in me at least two new ways:

1) There are supernatural physical changes occurring in the body *directly as a result of the power* now abiding in me, and

2) There are also physical changes happening because my will comprehends His will, and that causes me to act and to choose things that produce health.

Then he said, "No, I understand...*All things are working together for your good!"*

Isn't that awesome? That describes it *exactly!* That is what is happening! What great new revelation on that verse! And that is the perfect verse to describe how He is transfiguring me into His image! And, God so perfectly ties that in with our previous studies about love, in that *the reason* all things are finally working together for my good is because of the Kingdom truth in the Word, "to them that love God".

I have finally learned to place my love for God above all else in every area of my life, getting rid of the idols who used to hold first place. And there is also the Kingdom truth in the Word, "to them who are called according to His purpose". I am daily yielding and walking in the purpose He predestined in me before I was even born!

It is amazing to me the speed and depth at which He is leading you and me into deeper revelation of His Word! Each day we increase! In 1 Thessalonians 5:5 (NIV), we are told, "You are all sons of the light and sons of the day. We do not belong to the night or to the darkness." Beloved, Jesus came that we might have life and have it or more abundantly, some translations say "to the full". Isn't it time we partook of that provision?

The Word of God says in Romans 13:11-14 (NIV),

> And do this, understanding the present time.
> The hour has come for you to wake up
> from your slumber, because our salvation is
> nearer now than when we first believed.

> The night is nearly over; the day is almost here. So let us put aside the deeds of darkness and put on the armor of light.
>
> Let us behave decently, as in the daytime, not in orgies and drunkenness, not in sexual immorality and debauchery, not in dissension and jealousy.
>
> Rather, clothe yourselves with the Lord Jesus Christ, and do not think about how to gratify the desires of the sinful nature.

Beloved, I believe that this is the day, perhaps even the hour, of His soon return. One thing is for certain: we are closer than any other generation has been before. Now is the time to wake up! Get dressed! *Put on* the garment, the armor, of light and **clothe yourselves** with the Lord Jesus Christ. It is time to live in the fullness, the abundance, and the health His love hath provided, where *all* things work together for your good!

The Picture of Health® Daily Power Plan™

Day 84

Luke 12:34 (NIV)

> For where your treasure is, there your heart will be also.

Selah (pause and reflect)

Two days ago we looked at John 3:19, which says, "This is the verdict: Light has come into the world, but men *loved darkness instead of light* because their deeds were evil." We found also that it is written in John 12:46 that He has freely offered His Son, Jesus Christ, the light, to you **so that** <u>no one who believes in Him should stay in darkness</u>.

We learned that it is *love* (the source of His Glory, the light which is power) that activates your faith. In Galatians 5:6, we are taught that **faith *worketh* by love**. So, we discovered that the key to *comprehension* (revelation) of the power that worketh in you (and even the question as to whether it does work in you or not) ***depends on what it is that you love***.

That study and the next day after (from Romans 8:28) set my heart thinking on the scripture which is our devotional scripture for today. This text is found both in Luke 12:34 and Matthew 6:21 and returns us to the question: *What do we love most?*

Whatever you love most is what motivates your actions and your will.

When it is the Lord whom we love the most, when He has first place in our lives, Philippians 2:13 tells us, "…it is God who works in you to will and to act according to his good purpose."

As I read farther in Chapter 12 of the Gospel of Luke, it was hard for me to find a stopping point. Day after day, He leads us back to the same message, found throughout His Word! And, as we near the final weeks of our 100-day journey, the message, the passion, and the anointing of His Holy Spirit seem to be growing more intense and more powerful each day.

The message is undeniable for those who are listening: The Lord is drawing us to the revelation to prepare, to be ready, to lay hold of and possess the victory He purchased for us - spirit, soul, and body.

Why? First, because He paid the ultimate price in order to redeem us from the curse and from death, hell, and the grave and that price should no longer be taken for granted! And secondly, *so that* we can be the *living testimony* of His Glory to the world around us in this, the day of His return!

People in the world are desperate for hope and answers! Child of God, I cannot say this strongly enough! Christ, who is in us, is **the answer** they seek **and the hope** of glory! The real question is: Will they see Him in your life, *including your body?*

"Can't we just exclude the body, Michelle?" No. You are made in His image, Spirit, Soul, *and Body*. It is why He came in bodily form to pay the price for our complete redemption from sin.

Luke 6:44 declares, *"For every tree is known by his own fruit."* The body is the result (the fruit) of what the soul wills to act and to do. If you are truly led by the Spirit of God, if your love for Him is first place in your life, your body *will* reflect that because your choices will come from the mind renewed to the Word of God!

I challenge you today to ask yourself,

Is my life (even my body) a living testimony to the Lord and His power?

Do I stand ready and able to serve at any moment?

Mathew 3:8 (AMP) speaks of our fruit, telling us to "bring forth fruit that is consistent with repentance [let your lives prove your change of heart]", and Acts 26:20 says we should repent and turn to God and prove our repentance by our deeds.

In Luke 13:6-9 (NIV), Jesus told this parable, "A man had a fig tree, planted in his vineyard, and he went to look for fruit on it, but did not find any. So he said to the man who took care of the vineyard, 'For three years now I've been coming to look for fruit on this fig tree and haven't found any. Cut it down! Why should it use up the soil?' " 'Sir,' the man replied, 'leave it alone for one more year, and I'll dig around it and fertilize it. If it bears fruit next year, fine! If not, then cut it down.' "

In Mathew 7:17-20 (NIV), Jesus said, "Likewise every good tree bears good fruit, but a bad tree bears bad fruit. A good tree cannot bear bad fruit, and a bad tree cannot bear good fruit. Every tree that does not bear good fruit is cut down and thrown into the fire. Thus, by their fruit you will recognize them."

Yes, beloved, as we continue to stay steadfast in Him and make choices to glorify Him, it is by *our fruit we will be recognized* as the born-again, spirit-filled, magnificently-clothed-in-splendor Child of the Most High God!

The Picture of Health® Daily Power Plan™

Day 85

John 15:1-2 (The Message)

> I am the Real Vine and my Father is the Farmer. He cuts off every branch of me that doesn't bear grapes. And every branch that is grape-bearing he prunes back so it will bear even more.

Selah (pause and reflect)

Yesterday we talked about the fruit of our lives. We saw that Luke 6:44 declares, *"For every tree is known by his own fruit."* Today's verse takes this a bit further in looking at Christ's comparison of branches that produce fruit and those that do not.

Our scripture today brings out the point that God prunes off the branches that do not produce fruit, but He also prunes back the branches that do so that they might produce even more. I recently heard a speaker put it this way, "You are pruned if you do and pruned if you don't!"

The point is that in the walking out of divine health in your body, everyone will suffer a little in the flesh and in renewing the mind in order to be free or we will suffer in the flesh and in the mind because we remain in bondage. If you are going to suffer one way or the other, why not do the things that will produce the good result, the good fruit?

Disobedience and lack of self-control are what have messed up our lives.

Let's just be truthful. I am sure that is no real shocker to most of you. Many of you readily confess that you have no self-control. But I am here to tell you that it does not have to be that way. In fact, you were not even created for it to be that way!

Proverbs 25:28 says, "Like a city whose walls are broken down is a man who lacks self-control."

Luke 9:25 says, "What good is it for a man to gain the whole world, and yet lose or forfeit his very self?"

Romans 6:6 says, "For we know that our old self was crucified with him so that the body of sin might be done away with, that we should no longer be slaves to sin…"

And, 1 Corinthians 7:5 tells us that Satan will tempt you because of your lack of self-control!

Beloved, the scriptures from Galatians 5:19-21 list the acts of the sin nature and declare, "…I warn you, as I did before, that those who live like this will not inherit the kingdom of God."

But fear not! The deception that has kept you from the fullness of your inheritance is being bound up and cast out of our lives forever! You see, many have thought and believed that the weight of walking in self-control and obedience was completely on your shoulders. It is not! Let's just break that lie wide open here and now. This is not an issue of whether or not _you_ have enough will power.

As we read further in Galatians 5:22-23, the Word says,

> But the fruit _of the Spirit_ is love, joy, peace, patience, kindness, goodness, faithfulness, gentleness and self-control. Against such things there is no law.

The issue is power, but it is His power, not yours! Self-control comes from the Sprit of God. It is the fruit of the Holy Spirit. It is the evidence that you are His. (Remember? In Mathew 7:17-20, Jesus said, "Likewise every good tree bears good fruit, but a bad tree bears bad fruit.") To confess that you have no self-control is to confess that you are not of His tree. Oh! Oh! Oh! Eyes are popping open all over now!

As a Child of God, self-control does abide in you as the fruit of The Branch from the root of Jesse (Isaiah 11). The first two things you must do are repent of destructive words and change your confession about self-control! He invites you,

> "Live in me. Make your home in me just as I do in you. <u>In the same way that a branch can't bear grapes by itself but only by being joined to the vine, you can't bear fruit unless you are joined with me.</u>
>
> I am the Vine, you are the branches. When you're joined with me and I with you, the relation intimate and organic, *the harvest is sure to be abundant.*
>
> <u>Separated, you can't produce a thing</u>. Anyone who separates from me is deadwood, gathered up and thrown on the bonfire. But if you make yourselves at home with me and my words are at home in you, *you can be sure* that whatever you ask will be listened to and acted upon. This is how my Father shows who he is—when you produce grapes, **when you mature as my disciples.**"
>
> (John 15:4-8 The Message)
>
> (Emphasis added.)

THE PICTURE OF HEALTH®
DAILY POWER PLAN™
Day 86

Luke 12:43 (AMP)

> Blessed (happy and to be envied) is that servant whom his master finds so doing when he arrives.

Selah (pause and reflect)

Are ready for your wedding day? We have visited this topic several times now since beginning these daily walks with God. How is your progress coming? Have you let the truth from the Word of God penetrate into your choices in everyday life? Or, are you still procrastinating bringing your flesh under authority?

In Luke 12:35, Jesus is speaking to His disciples (*which are now you and me*). He says,

> Be dressed ready for service and keep your lamps burning, like men waiting for their master to return from a wedding banquet, **so that** when he comes and knocks they can *immediately* open the door for him.
>
> *It will be good for those servants whose master finds them watching when he comes.* I tell you the truth, he will dress himself to serve, will have them recline at the table and will come and wait on them.
>
> *It will be good for those servants whose master finds them ready,* even if he

comes in the second or third watch of the night. (Emphasis added.)

I will tell you once more, beloved, *now is the time* God is releasing His wellness revelation to the end-time Body of Christ. We must not be like the Pharisees who missed His first coming and the great reward!

The Lord is calling *us* up to a higher place of faithfulness and obedience, a place far away from the Pharisees. For our own protection, He instructs us in James 1:22, "Don't merely listen to the Word and so deceive yourselves! Do what it says!" And He reminds us in James 4:17 (NLT) "...it is sin to know what you ought to do and then not do it."

Some people foolishly kid themselves into thinking they are not rebellious; they think they have only "delayed obedience". The Master himself addresses this "delayed obedience" in the Scriptures from Luke, Chapter 12 (emphasis added). Here is what He has to say about it:

> "But suppose the servant says to himself, 'My master is taking a long time in coming,' and he then begins to beat the menservants and maidservants and *to eat and drink and get drunk*. The master of that servant will come *on a day when he does not expect him and at an hour he is not aware of.* He will cut him to pieces *and assign him a place with the unbelievers.*
>
> That servant *who knows his master's will and does not get ready or does not do what his master wants* will be beaten with many blows. But the one who does not know and does things deserving punishment will be beaten with few blows. *From everyone*

who has been given much, much will be demanded; and from the one who has been entrusted with much, much more will be asked.

I have come to bring fire on the earth, and how I wish it were already kindled!"

You cannot delay obedience indefinitely. There is a time coming when you will have no more days. The truth is you do not know when that day will be. If you did know, perhaps you would more promptly yield to His direction. For the Word says in Mathew 24:43 and Luke 12:39 (NIV), "But understand this: If the owner of the house had known at what hour the thief was coming, he would not have let his house be broken into."

Let me be very straightforward. It is far past time for death to stop stealing the life from the Children of Grace before their purpose is fulfilled!

Just last week I attended the funeral of a young man, just forty-six years old, who had literally dropped dead of a heart attack, in church, without any warning. In an instant he was gone. His family could take comfort knowing that he had just renewed his relationship with Christ in recent months and had partaken of communion just minutes before he died. But the great tragedy is that he should have lived another 70-80 years to proclaim the works and love of the Lord!

Yes, it is time for this to stop. But it will only stop when the children of God take their rightful authority over the enemy by living each day in willing obedience to the will of God the Father. This includes walking in wisdom and holiness in our physical bodies so that no door is left open for the enemy to enter in!

He has redeemed us from every sickness and every disease and every curse of the enemy (Galatians 3:13). He has given us a learned mind, knowledge, and wisdom for the asking. He has given us the power of the Holy Spirit and the Blood of Christ working in us. Whether we choose to receive and walk in that redemption or not depends *entirely* on us.

As you spend time with the Lord today, be challenged to repent for taking advantage of His grace, fix your thoughts on Him, and press toward the mark for the prize of the high calling of God in Christ Jesus!

In Christ, we do have the victory that overcomes the world. But you, beloved, must lay hold of it and make it your own! Blessed, happy, and to be envied is the one who does!

THE PICTURE OF HEALTH®
DAILY POWER PLAN™
Day 87

Proverbs 21:19-21 (NIV)

> In the house of the wise are stores of choice food and oil, but a foolish man devours all he has.

Proverbs 9:17-18 (NIV)

> "Stolen water is sweet; food eaten in secret is delicious!"

> But little do they know that the dead are there, that her guests are in the depths of the grave.

Selah (pause and reflect)

My friend, we'll call her D., related to me what has become one of my all time favorite illustrations. The company D. works for has a covered-dish fellowship once a month. She had successfully resisted having any dessert during the meal and ate "on plan" because she and several co-workers were faithfully attending *The Picture of Health*™ classes.

On the day in reference, everyone else had returned to his or her desks and D. was on clean-up duty. That's when it happened. She found herself alone in the kitchen with a pan of brownies! Yikes! She told me how she rapidly devoured several brownies before anyone else came in! She said, "I can't believe I did that!"

Another woman told me a similar story about having lunch with a friend. They were eating out and she had enjoyed a steak, salad, and steamed veggies. The restaurant had served fresh, hot yeast rolls, but she had easily declined them during the meal. However, after the meal, as the friend excused herself to the restroom, the woman found herself stuffing one roll after another in her mouth before the friend returned! She said,

"Why was I doing that?"

These women, like many other men and women through the ages, were still operating out of a mindset rooted in the fear of lack. At *The Picture of Health*™, we call it the "*slave mentality*". What does being a slave have to do with devouring brownies? *Trust.* Or more precisely, *distrust.*

This distrust, rooted in the fear of lack, can be seen as far back as the Israelites attitudes and behaviors in the wilderness after leaving Egyptian bondage. According to Exodus Chapter 8 and also Psalm 105:37 (KJV), God "…brought them forth *(out of slavery)* also with silver and gold: and there was not one feeble person among their tribes."

So when God brought them out of bondage, they were every one wealthy, healed, and free. (Note: This is a type and shadow, or a "picture", of our redemption in Christ.) What a miracle! The entire account in Exodus is an amazing witness to the power and love of God. But look what we see happening just after this magnificent deliverance (Exodus 16:2-3):

> In the desert the whole community grumbled against Moses and Aaron. The Israelites said to them, "If only we had died by the LORD's hand in Egypt! There we sat around pots of meat and ate all the food we wanted,

> but you have brought us out into this desert to starve this entire assembly to death."

Do they have a short-term memory problem? No, they (still) have a "*slave mentality*". Continue reading in Exodus 16:4-5 (emphasis added):

> Then the LORD said to Moses, "I will rain down bread from heaven for you. The people are to go out <u>each day</u> and gather <u>enough *for that day*</u>. In this way I will test them and see whether they will follow my instructions. On the sixth day they are to prepare what they bring in, and that is to be twice as much as they gather on the other days."

Skipping down to verse 19-20:

> Then Moses said to them, "No one is to keep any of it until morning."
>
> **However, some of them paid no attention to Moses; they kept part of it until morning**, but it was full of maggots and began to smell. So Moses was angry with them.

And then in verses 26-30 Moses commanded them *for the second time: (emphasis added)*

> "Six days you are to gather it, but on the seventh day, the Sabbath, there will not be any."
>
> *Nevertheless*, some of the people went out on the seventh day to gather it, but they found none. Then the LORD said to Moses, "*How long will you refuse to keep my commands and my instructions? Bear*

> *in mind that the LORD has given you the Sabbath; that is why on the sixth day he gives you bread for two days.* Everyone is to stay where he is on the seventh day; no one is to go out." So the people rested on the seventh day.

Why did they persist in this attitude of distrust and disobedience? Because they still held fast to the *"slave mentality",* a leftover mindset of fear, lack, distrust, and bondage. Very simply, <u>they had not renewed their mind</u>.

Years of thinking patterns, influenced by the Egyptian's world, made them resistant to accepting (believing, having faith in) the truth. God had not only been faithful to deliver them (as promised) from bondage, but He was also proving to be faithful in providing for them ***daily*** (also as promised). Some days He even provided twice as much so that they could have a day of rest! And, He provided all this while they were being disobedient! God is certainly long-suffering! Why? Because He wants His best for us whether we know that or not!

<u>Devouring brownies, or any other thing, is not so much about the brownies</u>

<u>as it is about forgetting our redemption through Christ!</u>

Relating this to our text from Proverbs 21, the fool feels the need to devour all the brownies because he fears that he might not get any more or he doesn't trust that he will have another opportunity to enjoy them. The real application of this is that he devours all he gets right away because he does not trust Christ as his Provider. This could be with brownies, or other foods or drink, but also with your finances, your relationships, etc.

A wise man, on the other hand, has stores of choice food and oil (or brownies) because he *trusts in God*. He does not fear the "missed opportunity" or "lack". He is no longer compelled to devour things quickly for momentary pleasure because he has no fear of never having them again. Yes, he can have a brownie anytime he wants. Led by the Spirit of God, he wisely chooses *when* to do so.

What keeps a wise man from being a glutton like the fool or like the Israelites in the desert? The mindset of *freedom*. The wise man knows that he can take his time, save or spend, eat or decline, feast or fast, as the Spirit leads. He is no longer a slave to compulsion because he trusts that God will always provide more than enough of everything needed for life and godliness.

2 Peter 1:3-9 says,

> His divine power has given us *everything* we need for **life** *and* **godliness** <u>through</u> our knowledge of him who called us by his own glory and goodness. Through these he has given us his very great and precious promises, **so that** through them you may *participate in the divine nature and escape the corruption in the world caused by evil desires.*
>
> For this very reason, make every effort to add to your *faith goodness*; and to goodness, *knowledge*; and to knowledge, *self-control*; and to self-control, *perseverance*; and to perseverance, *godliness*; and to godliness, brotherly *kindness*; and to brotherly kindness, *love*.

> For if you possess these qualities in increasing measure, *they will keep you from being ineffective and unproductive* in your knowledge of our Lord Jesus Christ.
>
> But if anyone does not have them, he is nearsighted and blind, and *has forgotten* that he has been cleansed from his past sins.

Beloved, are you still behaving like a slave in new clothes? Have you been delivered only to still walk in bondage? <u>Deliverance does not automatically bring freedom</u>. To fully *partake* of your deliverance, you must choose to accept – to believe - God's Word as Truth, renew your mind to it, and choose to operate in it.

As you finish your devoted time with God today, give great consideration to who He is. He is Jehovah Jireh - The Lord God who sees ahead and provides. Remember (don't forget) who you are through Him. Ask Him to show you thinking patterns that are keeping you trapped in slavery. Then, wash your mind with the Word, renewing it to walk in freedom!

THE PICTURE OF HEALTH®
DAILY POWER PLAN™
Day 88

John 6:12 (NIV)

> When they had all had enough to eat, he said to his disciples, "Gather the pieces that are left over. Let nothing be wasted."

<u>Selah (pause and reflect)</u>

Responding to His instructions to gather the pieces left over, the disciples gathered twelve baskets of food. The first and most often taught point of this is that the Lord will always provide, that it will be more than enough and then some.

But there is much more to it than that. Have you ever examined why he said "let nothing be wasted"? He isn't merely teaching on good stewardship, He was exposing a "heart condition".

After the miracle feeding of the multitudes, Jesus awoke the next day to find that the crowds had followed after him, even crossing the sea to find him. The interesting thing is that He rebuked them for doing so. Let's take some time to read this conversation from John 6:26-30 (NIV):

> Jesus answered, "I tell you the truth, you are looking for me, not because you saw miraculous signs but because you ate the loaves and had your fill. Do not work for food that spoils, but for food that endures to eternal life, which the Son of Man will give you. On

> him God the Father has placed his seal of approval."
>
> Then they asked him, "What must we do to do the works God requires?"
>
> Jesus answered, "The work of God is this: to believe in the one he has sent."
>
> So they asked him, "What miraculous sign then will you give that we may see it and believe you? What will you do?"

Jesus was teaching them about believing on Him and walking in faith. He was teaching them about the Kingdom of God, the Bread of Heaven, and eternal salvation; miracles, signs, and wonders were *following* His teaching to confirm the Word.

The people, however, had their minds fixed primarily on the works (what they could see and what else He would do for them). He fed them. He healed them. And still they asked, "What will you *do* that we might believe?" In verse 36, Jesus finally declared, "But as I told you, you have seen me and still you do not believe."

We can see a similar exchange in Malachi 1:10 (The Message) between the Lord and Israel, where the Lord said,

> Why doesn't one of you just shut the Temple doors and lock them? Then none of you can get in and play at religion with this silly, empty-headed worship. I am not pleased. The GOD-of-the-Angel-Armies is not pleased. And I don't want any more of this so-called worship!

Or, from the Amplified Version (emphasis added):

> Oh, that there were even one among you [whose duty it is to minister to Me] who would shut the doors, that you might not kindle fire on My altar to no purpose [*an empty, futile, fruitless pretense*]! I have no pleasure in you, says the Lord of hosts, nor will I accept an offering from your hand.

Here's the point: The crowd resisted learning to walk by faith. When He said, "Let nothing be wasted", perhaps He was showing them 'this is what comes by faith and you do not yet value it'. Jesus was exposing the condition of their hearts. Although they had *the appearance of seeking God*, their hearts were self-seeking, self-centered, and selfish. (Take note of how this *self*-interest is just another example of the slave mentality we spoke about yesterday!)

He perceived that they 'kindled fire' (followed him) in *empty, futile, fruitless pretense*. They wanted Him to do it for them. They wanted the provision and the miracles but did not desire true fellowship with Him.

Another place in the Bible this is addressed is in 2 Timothy 3:1-7 KJV (emphasis added):

> This know also, that in the last days perilous times shall come. For men shall be lovers of their own selves, covetous, boasters, proud, blasphemers, disobedient to parents, *unthankful, unholy*, without natural affection, trucebreakers, false accusers, incontinent, fierce, *despisers of those that are good*, traitors, heady, *highminded, lovers of pleasures more than lovers of God*;
>
> **Having a form of godliness, but denying the power thereof**: <u>from such turn away</u>. For

of this sort are they which creep into houses, and lead captive silly women laden with sins, led away with divers lusts,

<u>Ever learning, and never able to come to the knowledge of the truth.</u>

Daily as we walk with God, we should be those who judge ourselves and examine our hearts that we not be found *"ever learning, and never able to come to the knowledge of the truth"*, or *"having a form of godliness but denying the power thereof"*.

How do we do that? If you have been pretending to walk in faith, repent first and ask Him to guide you. Cease to treat the Lord's instruction as *casual*. Reverence what He has brought to you! Don't say one thing and do another. Find out what the Lord says and do it!

We can endeavor to be led by the Holy Spirit instead of our flesh. Let's do it. Let's be those who hearken to Him saying, "**<u>Let nothing be wasted</u>**."

The Picture of Health® Daily Power Plan™

Day 89

Romans 7:21-23 (NIV)

> So I find this law at work: When I want to do good, evil is right there with me. For in my inner being I delight in God's law; but I see another law at work in the members of my body, waging war against the law of my mind and making me a prisoner of the law of sin at work within my members.

Selah (pause and reflect)

Most people don't find it as easy to "prove yourself" or demonstrate that you are a Child of God as it is to say that you are one. Even among those whose hearts are genuinely for Him, there seems to remain a common perception that we sometimes lack the power to resist certain temptations.

For some of you it may be sweets or chocolate in times of stress. For others, it may be smoking, laziness, binging, eating in secret, or maybe resistance to exercise. Whatever your personal challenge is, we can all relate to Paul's grief at being "sold as a slave to sin" (Romans 7:14) and the perceived inability to break free from the "slave mentality".

For me, I'd have to say the greatest challenge has been to make exercise a priority. I used to hate exercise. I know it is good for me. I have done it for the past few years because I know it helps me to care for the temple of God, because it is what I teach to our weekly classes, and because it keeps me in shape to carry the Gospel. But to be honest, with multiple businesses to look after and a family of 13 and counting (including our three precious grandchildren), it has been a real effort to keep a good attitude and be consistent. That is until recently.

For the first time that I can remember, I *love* my workouts. I am up in the morning, ready to go. I am energized and excited about the changes I am seeing. My body is responding without as much effort. And my intensity and endurance have measurably improved. It isn't a burden anymore to exercise! What has happened?

You may remember that I began to feel this increase about Day 83 when I wrote to you about scripture in Romans 8:28, "all things working together for my good". That was quite a revelation in itself for me. But it has only gotten better since then! It has increased my hope, my joyful expectation, but also my performance of the actions that bring health to my body. It started one day as I studied for our time together. I heard Him speak, not audibly but to my heart,

"This is not about you."

This is additional revelation about the rest of the verse from Romans 8:28: "for those who are called *according to His purpose*". This, meaning "my life", is not about me. Neither is yours.

As the truth continued to sink in over the next few days, I heard my pastor say, "God was not created for you, but rather you were created for Him." The Lord had led me even deeper into what I know in my life has been true breakthrough revelation!

Let's tie this back in to our discussion about the conflict between your desires and your actions. When we are self-centered rather than God-centered, the power to overcome seems to lie within our own ability or the lack thereof as the case might be. The truth, however, is that for the Believer, our ability is now irrelevant. Follow this through the scriptures:

When God created man and woman, the Bible tells us:

> It was "for *thy pleasure* they are and were created" (Revelation 4:11 KJV),
>
> "for *His glory*" (Isaiah 43:7)
>
> to *do good works,* which He prepared in advance for you *to do* (Ephesians 2:10),
>
> "for the *praise of His glory*" (Ephesians 1:12),
>
> to be like God in righteousness and holiness (Ephesians 4:24),
>
> and for "*fellowship with Him*", a holy people of His very own. (Titus 2:14).

But…when sin came into the world, sin separated us all from God (Isaiah 59:2). Man became self-centered and self-conscious (Genesis 3:8), sacrificing his God-created purpose for momentary pleasure. But that's not all. What I would like you to see today is that we were *separated from our purpose*, the very reason we were created!

As a result of choosing sin, we no longer were in fellowship; we no longer brought Him glory or caused men to praise Him; our lives bore a curse and ceased to be a testimony of His glorious provision. Not because He desired it, but because man chose it. God didn't diminish, nor did He stop loving us. His Righteousness demanded just consequence. Separation and death are the consequence of sin.

> But now he has reconciled you by Christ's physical body through death to present you holy in his sight, without blemish and free from accusation— (Colossians 1:22 NIV)

That is what **is** about you, beloved. *The Cross of Christ is about you*. All your faults, weaknesses of the flesh, struggles, and sin debt were taken by Christ on the Cross; He was crucified to redeem you from them.

> You see, at just the right time, when we were still powerless, Christ died for the ungodly. (Romans 5:6)

> But God demonstrates his own love for us in this: While we were still sinners, Christ died for us. (Romans 5:8)

> For what I received I passed on to you as of first importance: that Christ died for our sins according to the Scriptures… (1 Corinthians 15:3)

Glory to God! Do you see this? The Cross is all about you because of His love for you! Redeeming you. Reconciling you. Restoring you. Yes, beloved, *the Cross was about you*.

Romans 8:1 (NIV) says, "Therefore, there is now no condemnation for those who are in Christ Jesus". If you are still trapped in the struggle, habits of the flesh, or buried emotions, you are not operating "*in* Christ". You are still operating in the "old man". Accepting His death on the cross as payment for your life means acknowledging that you died with Him and all your selfish actions and desires were nailed there and buried there.

Jesus said in Luke 14:27 & 33 (AMP),

> Whoever does not persevere and carry his own cross and come after (follow) Me cannot be My disciple.
>
> ...any of you who does not forsake (renounce, surrender claim to, give up, say good-bye to) all that he has cannot be My disciple.

Beloved, if you are still crying out for God to do it for you, to take away the persecution or the temptation, you need to *go back to the Cross* and examine what was accomplished there!

In all love, beloved, I tell you: the Cross was about you BUT... as He died for you, Jesus proclaimed,

"It is finished."

Just as He said it to my heart, I believe He is speaking to us all from that statement. Life is not just about you anymore. Get past it. Now it is time to accept, believe, and have faith in who you are ***in Him*** and move on to the reason you were redeemed.

THE PICTURE OF HEALTH®
DAILY POWER PLAN™
Day 90

2 Corinthians 9:13 (New International Version)

> Because of the service by which you have proved yourselves, men will praise God for the obedience that accompanies your confession of the gospel of Christ, and for your generosity in sharing with them and with everyone else.

Selah (pause and reflect)

Ever thought much about that? Will men praise God for the obedience that accompanies your confession of the Gospel of Christ? Are people led to Christ as much by the witness of your life, including the condition of your body, as they are by the words you say to them? Is there anything for others to see, past you, that draws them to Christ?

I heard a story several years ago about the death of Daisy Osborne, one of God's great missionaries and women of faith. It was said to me that when she died, a friend reflected that Daisy hadn't really died that day, but that Daisy had died years ago.

As I read about her life and ministry at her husband's side, I came to understand that it truly was no longer Daisy who lived, but Christ in her. As a student in Bible school, studying in the very building that she and T.L. Osborne built for the Lord, I determined I wanted a life like that, a legacy like that for my children to inherit.

Even though she has long ago moved to heaven, her testimony has stayed with me all these years. I am learning that it is not without cost in the natural; things, seemingly precious things, are given up in order to live for and *in Him*. Yet, when it seems difficult to follow through in the natural, I remember Daisy and I am strengthened by the truth that her daily decision, and the decision of many like her, was to live as Christ. These decisions were of eternal consequence in the lives of literally millions of people. Even in her physical death, men and women worldwide praised God for the obedience that accompanied her confession of the Gospel of Christ.

Beloved, our lives are to be no different. Look at this: (note the emphasis added)

> Now <u>if we died with Christ</u>, we believe that <u>we will also live with him</u>. (Romans 6:8 NIV)

> So, my brothers, you also died to the law through the body of Christ, that <u>you might belong to another, *to him*</u> who was raised from the dead, <u>in order that ***we might bear fruit to God***</u>. (Romans 7:4 NIV)

> Since <u>you died with Christ</u> to the basic principles of this world, why, as though you still belonged to it, do you submit to its rules? (Colossians 2:20 NIV)

> For <u>you died</u>, and <u>your life is now hidden with Christ *in* God</u>. (Colossians 3:3 NIV)

> For this reason Christ is the mediator of a new covenant, *that those who are called may receive the promised eternal inheritance—*

> now that he has died as a ransom to set them free from the sins committed under the first covenant. (Hebrews 9:15 NIV)
>
> For Christ died for sins once for all, the righteous for the unrighteous, *to bring you to God*. He was put to death in the body but made alive by the Spirit, (1 Peter 3:18 NIV)

Let's look at Romans 6:6-10 (NIV) (note the emphasis added):

> For we know that <u>our old self *was* crucified with him</u> *so that* the body of sin might be done away with, <u>that we should no longer be slaves</u> to sin— because anyone who has died **has been** freed from sin.
>
> Now if we died with Christ, we believe that we will also ***live with him***. For we know that since Christ was raised from the dead, he cannot die again; death no longer has mastery over him.
>
> ***<u>The death he died, he died to sin once for all</u>***; but ***<u>the life he lives, he lives to God</u>***.

This is what God meant when He said to me, "It is not about you."

If when we receive Christ as Savior, *we died with Christ* and believe we live with Him, and the Word of God tells us that the life Christ lives <u>He lives to God</u>, then, beloved, we now should be living unto God.

That's right! The old man is passed away. Your new, *redeemed* life is wholly about being "called according to *His* purpose" (Romans 8:28). Can you see this? Christ reconciled you to God *so that* <u>your purpose</u>, your original purpose, could be fulfilled!

Do you remember that purpose? We identified it in the Word yesterday. It is to live ***<u>in Him</u>***, bringing glory to Him, for fellowship with Him, and most of all, to be witnesses of Him! Before ascending to heaven, Christ commissioned all Believers to *be witnesses*, going to all the world, preaching and teaching the Kingdom of God, the Gospel of Christ, and healing the sick in His Name.

Beloved, that is what our lives are to be about now. Make a heart change today. You are equipped to do this. It is written in Philippians 2:13, "for it is God who works in you to will and to act according to his good purpose." You just have to decide, be willing, and speak His Truth.

<u>Be witnesses</u> of the love and power of God
to the world today.

THE PICTURE OF HEALTH®
DAILY POWER PLAN™
Day 91

James 4:10 (New Living Translation)

> When you bow down before the Lord and admit your dependence on him, he will lift you up and give you honor.

Selah (pause and reflect)

For the past few days, we have been discovering the truth from the Word of God that once you receive Christ as Savior, the purpose of your health journey, like everything else in your life, should be about glorifying God and presenting *a living witness of the Gospel* to others.

Today, let's examine how that directly relates to your health journey and the challenges you might face today. The first truth is:

> *You were helpless before the cross.*
> *You are not helpless now.*

The desires of your flesh were crucified on the cross, you died with Him, and …here's what you need to know now: You rose with Him too! You have the power, the keys to the Kingdom of Heaven. If you are still crying out for Him to take things from you, you need to take one last look at the cross, tell your old self, "Goodbye!" and move on into the resurrected power of His Glory!

To "carry your cross daily" is to remember that your old self and your old selfish purposes *are crucified and dead*. You are now a new creation raised in power to new life!

Make your everyday actions be those in which His power is exalted in your life. When you do, others will marvel at His strength at work in you and want to know about it! That is being His witness. That is living as Christ, on purpose.

As we comprehend that living healthy is about **how others will see Him** *(not us)*, we can operate in the confidence that He who began a good work in us will carry it on to completion until the day of Christ's return (Philippians 1:6).

For too many years, children of Grace have misused or misinterpreted this precept, mistaking 'dependence on Him' with 'helplessness'. Bowing down is an act of submission…*not helplessness*. You were helpless *before* the cross. You are *not* helpless now.

Notice it says, "When you bow down". That is an action. It takes discipline and obedience to "bow down", to submit. Look at it this way: it isn't submission if you agree or if you want to do it. It only becomes submission when you would rather do it another way (or not at all!).

Submission is a deliberate act of choosing to honor God.

Think of Christ in the Garden. As a natural man, he would rather have had the cup of torture and death pass from him. We know that from the scriptures. Yet, because He so loved God… and you, He prayed for the will of God to be done. Do you think that was easy? No. But God's Grace answered Jesus' prayer and empowered him to endure it!

Was it worth it? Every soul that receives the gift of eternal life is evidence that it was. Remember the story I told you of Daisy Osborne? All the lives I will touch with God's love and truth are in part a result of her life lived *in Him*.

The legacy or inheritance *you* leave behind is no less important *if* that legacy is a life *lived in Him*. In the same way He empowered Christ to go to the cross, His grace empowers you. But, beloved, you are the one who must choose to bow down. You must be willing, in the same way Christ was willing, to carry the cross, to die to self, for the greater purpose of exalting Him! Therein is found the grace to endure.

> Here is a trustworthy saying:
>
> If we died with him,
>
> we will also live with him;
>
> if we endure,
>
> we will also reign with him.
>
> If we disown him,
>
> he will also disown us;
>
> if we are faithless,
>
> he will remain faithful,
>
> for he cannot disown himself.
>
> 2 Timothy 2:11-13 (NIV)

THE PICTURE OF HEALTH®
DAILY POWER PLAN™
Day 92

Colossians 2:9-10 (Amplified Bible)

> For in Him the whole fullness of Deity (the Godhead) continues to dwell in bodily form [giving complete expression of the divine nature].
>
> And you are in Him, made full and having come to fullness of life [in Christ you too are filled with the Godhead—Father, Son and Holy Spirit—and reach full spiritual stature]. And He is the Head of all rule and authority [of every angelic principality and power].

Selah (pause and reflect)

Beloved, this is what we have been grasping, little by little, precept upon precept, for these past 91 days. It is the renewing of our minds to the truth of who we are ***In Him***. Colossians 2:10 tells us that we are complete in Him. And He is the head of all principalities and power.

To continue from yesterday, my questions to you is, "If you are in Him, who, then, are you in relation to principalities and powers?" We learned yesterday that we are not helpless when we are ***in Him***. What else? What other truths can we lay hold of? What more has He made available to strengthen us, and our actions, according to the power that worketh in us?

When we began this journey together, I prayed for you from Ephesians that the eyes of your understanding would be opened to know Him better. Let's take a short survey of Colossians to highlight some powerful verses that will further open our eyes to our glorious inheritance through Christ. It is through that inheritance that Believers live and move and have their being (Acts 17:28)! It is *in Him* that we have every victory!

According to the Word of God, ***in Him*** ...

...you are the image of the invisible God, the brightness of His glory and the express image of His person (Colossians 1:15, Genesis 1:27, Phil 2:6, Heb 1:3).

...you were created by Him, for Him, that in you should all fullness dwell (Colossians 1:16, 1:19)

...you are reconciled and presented to the Lord holy, unblameable, and unreproveable in His sight (Colossians 1:22).

...you are complete, buried with Him in baptism, risen with Him through faith, rooted and built up in Him. In Him you are established (confirmed, made sure) in every good work. (Colossians 2:7,10,12)

He has quickened your flesh, your mortal body (Psalm 119:50, Psalm 119:93,1 Corinthians 15:36, Ephesians 2:1, Ephesians 2:5, Colossians 2:13, 1 Peter 3:18,Romans 8:11).

> (Note: from Strong's Concordance, to quicken means to: cause to live; make alive; give life by spiritual power; to arouse and invigorate; to restore to life; to give increase of life: thus of physical life)

In accepting Christ as Savior, you have put on a new man (Spirit, Soul, and Body) after the image of He who created you (Colossians 3:10).

Why do I bring these things out to you today? What do these things have to do with your health journey? Everything.

Every good and perfect blessing from the Father is found *in Him*. These truths are the Word of God, who is Christ. In Him, who is The Word, *and only in Him*, will you will find the desires of your heart, health for your flesh and strength for your bones! (Proverbs 3:8, 16:24)

THE PICTURE OF HEALTH®
DAILY POWER PLAN™
Day 93

Ephesians 4:11-13 (King James Version) *italics added for emphasis*

> And he gave some, apostles; and some, prophets; and some, evangelists; and some, pastors and teachers;
>
> For the perfecting of the saints, for the work of the ministry, for the edifying of the body of Christ:
>
> Till we all come in *the unity of the faith*, and of the knowledge of the Son of God, *unto a perfect man*, unto the measure of the stature of the *fulness of Christ*:

Selah (pause and reflect):

"*Unto a perfect man*". Wow. What a goal! Is that even do-able? Many have tried. The Lord knows I did for more than thirty years! As I look through the Word, I find that I was in good company. The Apostle Paul spoke of "pressing on toward the goal" in Philippians 3:12. He wrote, "Not that I have already obtained all this, or have already been made perfect, but I press on to take hold of that for which Christ Jesus took hold of me."

But is it do-able? Can we truly reach that perfection? The answer is yes…and no. No, you alone cannot reach that goal. But, yes, all things are possible with God. No, you cannot be flawless or without mistake. But, yes, you can be perfect. *How's that?*

If you look at Paul's life, you will find it much like many of ours. For years he attempted to reach "perfection" (and please God) by the world's definition of the word. For years, he moved further and further from the goal. Then somewhere along the road to Damascus, he was mercifully blinded to the enemy's deception and saw clearly for the first time the Lord's true desire and definition of perfection.

You see, Strong's Concordance identifies the Word used for "perfect" in Ephesians 4:13 as the Greek word "teleios" {tel'-i-os}, which means "that which is brought to its end, finished, or wanting nothing necessary to *completeness*". In short, it means to **grow up**!

Ephesians 4:14-15 says when we are made *perfect (meaning grown up in Christ),* "then we *will no longer be infants, tossed back and forth by the waves, and blown here and there* by every wind of teaching and by the cunning and craftiness of men in their deceitful scheming. Instead, speaking the truth in love, we will *in all things* grow up into him who is the Head, that is, Christ."

Are you ready for the scales of deception to be loosed from your eyes and to see clearly, perhaps for the first time ever, the Lord's true definition of perfection? Are you longing to stop being blown here and there by every wind of teaching on how to regain and retain your physical health? How about this: Are you ready to receive the perfect, healed, complete body that Christ died to redeem for you?

Ephesians 4:15, says that by *"speaking the truth in love,* we will *in all things* grow up into him who is the Head, that is, Christ." That is what I am endeavoring to do with you from the Word in these last several days. For today, I leave you with these thoughts to consider:

Hebrews 11:24 (NIV) tell us that *"By faith* Moses, when he had grown up, *refused to be known as* the son of Pharaoh's daughter." You have a choice, like Moses had, that you must make by faith. The Pharaoh's daughter represented the worldly kingdom and its ways. Moses chose to leave it by faith. He made a grown-up decision not to be known as the world's child any longer.

The fullness of His redemption is a gift to you. It remains your choice as to whether you receive it or not. It is your decision to make as to whose child you will be known as.

THE PICTURE OF HEALTH®
DAILY POWER PLAN™
Day 94

Hebrews 5:12 (King James Version)

> For when for the time ye ought to be teachers, ye have need that one teach you again which be the first principles of the oracles of God; and are become such as have need of milk, and not of strong meat.

Selah (pause and reflect):

It was a hot, 120-degree day in August when our furnishings were delivered to Mexico. We were new missionaries, in a foreign country, no toilet, no doors, hundreds of giant roaches and scorpions for house companions, and that is the better side of the picture! Oh, yes, and there was also that mouse and large pile of doggie poop to welcome me on the very first night.

I thought I was ready. After all, I had been to Bible School and World Missions Training! I had taken months to prepare and had come equipped. That is, until I had the "meltdown". In the context of our scripture above, I "choked"! My parents, who had moved us out of the country and into Mexico, came over to say their goodbyes and I crumbled. They had two words of wisdom for me as they drove off… **"Grow up."**

That was it. They were gone and the moving truck with them. It was too late to turn back now! According to Proverbs 13:13 (MSG), I then had two options: "Ignore the Word and suffer; honor God's commands and grow rich."

In other words, I could continue to be "tossed about to and fro" or I could be a doer of the Word of God and grow up!

Well, I reasoned, being "tossed about" was not producing pleasing results, and I was thousands of miles from my comfort zone, so, I chose to grow up. I cut off my hair (so the roaches wouldn't land in it) and I pressed in to God for strength and I moved forward in His divine purpose for my life. It wasn't easy but it was just that simple. And His grace was sufficient. It was the best and worst year of my life. But I grew. It was the *real* start of my equipping for the work of the ministry. It was the beginning of the path that led me to you!

My pastor recently commented that…

There is no such thing as a spiritual giant who is an emotional basket case.

So true! I mused at that thought, quickly recalling the story I just shared with you. I am thankful for my mother's wisdom, for the lessons God taught me on the mission field, for the much wiser missionaries He surrounded me with, and for the seeds of His Word that were planted that *continue* to grow me up today.

But then, as I chuckled at my thoughts and my own immaturity, I was challenged by another thought, an equally powerful truth from the Lord:

Nor is there a spiritual giant who is a <u>physical</u> basket case.

My thoughts went to the billions of Christians, even to many leaders, who are "tossed back and forth" in their weight or by one disease after another, tormented by the physical results of their childish, carnal ways. I knew once more why we are called and chosen to do what we do.

We left Mexico one year after that scorching hot day in August. We were disappointed to leave the people we had come to love so dearly and the service in the Kingdom that was so rewarding. But it was time for another growing up season. My husband inquired of the Lord as to why He was calling us home and the Lord's reply was from 1 Thessalonians 5:23 (NIV), "May God himself, the God of peace, sanctify you through and through. May your *whole spirit, soul and body* be kept blameless at the coming of our Lord Jesus Christ." And from Ephesians 4 (our "Power Verse" for yesterday), "For the *perfecting of the saints, for the work of the ministry, for the edifying of the body of Christ…*" (Italics are mine.)

The Lord ministered to our hearts that His Body (us included) was "sicker than the world and it should not be so". We came to understand that millions of children of God were missing out on the full measure of the fullness in Christ and dying before their "expected end". He promised our hearts that if we would be willing and obedient, be teachable, and seek Him first, He would reveal to us the great mystery of His Word, that He would show us the Way, the Truth, and the Life that would deliver His people from the deception of the enemy.

So there you have it! That is how we came to "walk" with you today! That is how this daily devotional was birthed. It is His Word ministering to you, in love, so that you can reach "the measure of the stature of the fulness of Christ", your "*full spiritual stature*" **in Him**. (Ephesians 4:13, Colossians 2:10)

I'll leave you with one more scripture about growing up. It is what God said to me back then and it is still what He is saying to each of us now:

> "In a word, what I'm saying is, Grow up. You're kingdom subjects. Now live like it. Live out your God-created identity. Live generously and graciously toward others, the way God lives toward you."
>
> Matthew 5:48 (The Message)

THE PICTURE OF HEALTH®
DAILY POWER PLAN™
Day 95

Ephesians 3:9 (Young's Literal Translation) *italics added for emphasis*

> *…to cause all to see what [is] the fellowship of the secret that hath been hid from the ages in God*, who all things did create by Jesus Christ…

<u>*Selah (pause and reflect)*</u>:

Remember when we learned that we are made in His image? It was back on Day 52, from Genesis 1:26-27. We learned that there is, by design, an inseparable union (communion) between our Spirit, Soul, and Body. Then, on Day 77 and others, we received revelation from the Word on "the power that worketh in us". Did you notice that our scripture text today uses both of these Kingdom principles together?

In those previous days, we saw in the Word that our three parts, like His three parts (Father, Son, and Holy Spirit) are three-in-one, all unique but never functioning completely independent of one another, but instead, they are in constant and continual communication with each other. We learned that the Greek word for this Kingdom principle is "*koinonia*" (koy-nohn-ee'-ah).

Searching the Scriptures, I found that "koinonia" occurs twenty (20) times in eighteen (18) verses in the Word of God. "Koinonia" means fellowship (in the text above), joint participation, communication, and intercourse. It expresses the characteristic not simply of unity or casual relationship, but that of a much more established and powerful *intimacy* or *intimate union*.

The concept and power of "koinonia" can be seen in Jesus' words from John 17:21-23 (KJV) *(emphasis added is mine)*:

> That they all **may be one; as thou, Father, art in me, and I in thee**, that they also may be **one in us**: *that the world may believe that thou hast sent me.*
>
> And the glory which thou gavest me *I have given them*; **that they may be one, even as we are one:**
>
> **I in them, and thou in me**, that they **may be made perfect in one**; and *that the world may know that thou hast sent me, and hast loved them, as thou hast loved me.*

Do you see the desire of His heart? It is the message from the Word that the Lord is breathing throughout the earth in these days. In the wind of the Holy Spirit is His end-time revelation, the revelation of the great mystery. As we reach for the final harvest, the operation of this Kingdom force is to be *the evidence of the Father's love* for the world, for us, and for you.

THE PICTURE OF HEALTH®
DAILY POWER PLAN™
Day 96

Isaiah 59:2a (New International Version)

> But your iniquities have separated you from your God;

Selah (pause and reflect):

Now, think back (or look back) to our study on Day 89 where we studied *why* we were created. We saw in the Word that it was "for [God's] pleasure" (Revelation 4:11 KJV) and for "*fellowship with Him*", a holy people of His very own (Titus 2:14). I found that the Word says in Genesis, chapter 3, that God created the Garden of Eden especially for man to live in, a place where God and man could walk together in the "cool of the day". As I studied this out, I began to see it, as I hope you are now beginning to…

Constant, intimate fellowship was His desire and design from the beginning!

But wait! Before you too readily agree, notice that His intent for this "fellowship" was not like the relationship we commonly mistake it for, nor was it to describe the mere gathering of friends or acquaintances. No, no, no. To understand this perfectly (more completely) and thereby to know how much deeper and infinitely more powerful His love is for us, we have to explore this beyond what we, the Body of Christ as a whole, have previously known or recognized and preached since His resurrection! So, stay hooked! I promise for those who decide to have eyes to see, you will be blessed beyond measure!

This fellowship is defined as "communion" or "intercourse". It is also defined as "communication", as in the vehicle He uses to express His love (like in the marriage union between man and wife). But, taking it even further, *within the communication or fellowship exists the very source, the power, the force, by which man's every need and desire can be satisfied.*

Remember! Man was created *for this very purpose*. He was created *for* fellowship with God. Man's spirit was created for it. Man's soul was created for it. And man's physical body was created for it. Man's authority over the earth and its inhabitants and the power to rule and reign were both a result of this fellowship, this "abiding communion". Man's very purpose was fulfilled in it and through it. Everything in man's life, all that he knew, was good because of it. (Wow. *Selah*.)

But…Ephesians 3:10-12 (NIV) tells us it was God's intent and "eternal purpose" that we not only be able to approach Him with confidence, but also with **freedom**. To establish that freedom, God gave man a command *and* choice. The Lord set man in the Garden and gave him access to everything with one exception: He commanded him not to eat of the tree of the knowledge of good and evil or he would surely die.

Being deceived by the serpent, Eve ate of the tree and also did Adam. Together they exercised that freedom of choice and in Genesis 3:23 we see that it cost them their relationship with God. Romans 5:12-20 (NIV) says that "sin entered the world through one man, and death through sin…", "and in this way death came to all men", that "judgment followed one sin and brought condemnation". Their actions did not just affect Adam and Eve, but by "the disobedience of the one man the many were made sinners".

(Side comment: Perhaps that is new to you if you do not yet know Christ as Savior. It is the key to understanding your need, every man's need, for redemption. But, the Good News is on the way for you so don't leave now! On the other hand, if you have been in Christ for some time, this may sound elementary to you. If that's you, you don't leave now either, for **you** just might be especially surprised at where this is going!)

Bring your focus back to the physical body for just a minute. These daily devotions are called "power walks" because they are designed to "exercise your faith and build *your body*™". The Kingdom principle we are examining in these last days is a vital key to understanding why so many in the Body of Christ are still sick and struggling in their physical bodies! It is why, although healing was purchased by Christ at the cross (Isaiah 53:5), Christians can't get well and stay well. It is why they can't seem to lose excess weight or gain it, which ever applies, or have authority over their carnal flesh. It is the answer to finally overcoming whatever physical challenges brought you to this book in the first place.

People come up with all kinds of *explanations and speculations and excuses* as to why Christians are sick or, more directly, why *they* are sick. Some say it is just the way they were born or it is "hereditary". Others say it is just how God made them to be, still believing that it may be God's will for some people to be sick or suffer or be overweight, etc. Some say it is to teach one a lesson of some kind. Some say it is just because we live on the earth. Some say it is because the sick person doesn't have enough faith. Still others say it is a sign of sinful living.

But what does *the Word* say?

Will you believe it? It says *none of the above*! Here is the truth from the Word of God: When death came into the earth <u>as a result of the sin</u> of Adam and Eve, it was called the "curse" (Genesis, chapter 3). All manner of sickness and disease of any and every kind is part of the curse (Deuteronomy, chapter 28). Man's earthly body began to die when man disobeyed God because that is what God told Adam would be the consequences for eating of the fruit of that tree (Genesis, chapter 2). This is *why* sickness and disease and imperfection in the body, and in the world, began. But the question still yet to be asked by the majority of those in the Body of Christ for all these years is…

What was it about sin that caused it to result in death?

The Word says in the beginning text of Isaiah 59:2 that:

Sin separated us <u>*from God.*</u>

That is the primary reason God did not want man to sin… because He is holy and in Him there is no – and could be no "intimate union" with- sin! He *is* life. He *is* light. In Him is (and could be) *no darkness at all* (1 John 1:5).

I hope you see it. Man could no longer remain in communion (where the source of life and all things necessary for life existed) because sin was in him; he could no longer remain in the holy presence of God and live. He would either die an immediate death in the garden right there in front of the Glory, or, God, in His mercy, had to banish man from His presence.

I really laid that foundation to get to this deeper truth: it wasn't only the sin that brought death but the sin *and* the resulting separation, which *moved us out of the provision of life!* God decreed that if Man ate of the tree of the knowledge of good and evil they would die. He did not lie nor did He change. Banishment (separation) in itself brought death, albeit eventual rather than immediate, but still death, to the natural body *because*...I said, *because*... communion with the supernatural life force had been severed! (That's found in Ephesians 4:18). From that point forward man was subject to the life span available in the natural. And, because the curse also came on the earth itself, as the earth began to die, that natural life span decreased generation by generation.

So! That explains it! That is why people are sick! *Wrong.* It only explains *why the world is, or the nations are, sick.* And, sin and separation explained how Old Testament Jews might have been sick. But that still doesn't explain why New Testament Believers, who are the Redeemed of the Lord, are still sick! ***Or does it?*** We'll look at that tomorrow!

THE PICTURE OF HEALTH®
DAILY POWER PLAN™

Day 97

1 John 1:6-7 (New International Version)

> If we claim to have fellowship with him yet walk in the darkness, we lie and do not live by the truth.
>
> But if *we* walk in the light, as *he* is in the light, we have *fellowship* one with another, and the blood of Jesus Christ his Son cleanseth us from all sin.

Selah (pause and reflect):

We finished up our "walk" yesterday discovering why *the world* suffers sickness, disease, and lack. We learned that it wasn't only because of the sin that brought death into the world, but also the resulting separation from God, which *moved all mankind out of the provision of life*!

But is it the same for *Christians* as it is for the world?

The short answer is no, it is not the same. However, to really comprehend why Christians are still suffering sickness, disease, and lack, we must first comprehend *and believe* the Word about the things that *do not* cause them to suffer sickness, disease, and lack.

For example, unlike the world, Christians are not sick because of sin. They are not sick because of the consequences of sin. They are not even sick because they are separated from God. They are not sick because of the curse. And, they are not sick because of genetics! *(Surprised?)*

How can I say this with such absolute certainty? Because I am fully persuaded by the Word.

First, if you are a Christian, then The Word says your sins have been paid for:

> Whom God hath set forth to be a propitiation through faith in his blood, to declare his righteousness ***for the remission of sins*** that are past, through the forbearance of God; (Romans 3:25 KJV)

> And ***he is the propitiation for our sins***: and not for ours only, *but also for the sins of the whole world.* (1 John 2:2 KJV)

> Herein is love, not that we loved God, but that he loved us, and sent his Son to be ***the propitiation for our sins***. (1 John 4:10 KJV)

Next, when Christ died for our sins and was resurrected in Glory, we were reconciled from the separation which brought death in. It is written (italics mine):

> But now he has ***reconciled* you** by Christ's physical body through death to present you holy in his sight, without blemish and free from accusation… (Colossians 1:22 NIV)

Additionally, regarding the curse (Deuteronomy, chapter 28) which brought every form of sickness and disease upon the world, Galatians 3:13 (NIV) says (emphasis added):

> **Christ redeemed us from the curse** of the law by becoming a curse for us, for it is written: "Cursed is everyone who is hung on a tree." He redeemed us in order that the

> blessing given to Abraham might come to the Gentiles through Christ Jesus, so that by faith we might receive the promise of the Spirit.

And further, in the Word from Romans we see that:

> Again, the gift of God is not like the result of the one man's sin: The judgment followed one sin and brought condemnation, but <u>*the gift followed many trespasses and brought justification*</u>. (Romans 5:16 NIV)

> Therefore, <u>*there is now no condemnation for those who are in Christ*</u> Jesus (Romans 8:1 NIV)

These passages from the Word tell us clearly that Christians should not suffer sickness, disease, and lack because we have been fully, completely redeemed from it! Come on now! See it with your Spirit! He desires *"that ye may be in strength to comprehend*, with all the saints, <u>what [is] the breadth, and length, and depth, and height,</u> *to know also the love* of the Christ *that is **exceeding the knowledge***, that ye may be *filled — to all the fulness of God"*. Ephesians 3:18-19 (YLT)

He wants you to comprehend the width, length, depth, and height of His will, His design, His desire, His Redemption, *His Great Mystery,* to exceed the (ordinary) knowledge so that we can come into the fullness of the full measure in Christ! The great mystery is that the fullness, the full measure is available **now** *In Christ*.

**When we were reconciled through Christ,
He accomplished the restoration**

of *fellowship, communion, life-giving intercourse,*

with the Lord God, Jehovah Elohim.

Selah.

THE PICTURE OF HEALTH®
DAILY POWER PLAN™

Day 98

Philippians 3:10-11 (Amplified Bible) *Emphasis added.*

> *[For my determined purpose is]* that I may know Him [that I may *progressively* become *more deeply and intimately acquainted* with Him, perceiving and recognizing and understanding the wonders of His Person more strongly and more clearly], and that I may *in that same way* come to know the power outflowing from His resurrection [which it exerts over believers], and *that I may so share His sufferings as to be continually transformed* [in spirit into His likeness even] to His death, [in the hope] That if possible I may attain to the [spiritual and moral] resurrection [that lifts me] out from among the dead *[even while in the body]*.

<u>*Selah (pause and reflect)*</u>:

Did you do that after our "power walk" yesterday? Did you "Selah", pause and reflect? To miss this is to miss the greatest love, the greatest compassion, ever expressed.

God's great mystery is being revealed. Down through the ages it has been hidden in the depths of The Word, waiting for such a time as this. (See Romans 16:25, Colossians 1:26, Ephesians 3:9, Ephesians 1:9) Behold the Truth from the Word of God:

> This is a profound **mystery** - but I am talking about Christ and the church. (Ephesians 5:32 NIV)
>
> I do not want you to be ignorant of this **mystery**, brothers, so that you may not be conceited: Israel has experienced a hardening in part *until* the full number of the Gentiles has come in. (Romans 11:25 NIV)
>
> To them God has chosen to make known among the Gentiles <u>*the glorious riches*</u> of this **mystery**, which is Christ <u>*in you*</u>, the hope of <u>*glory*</u>. (Colossians 1:27 NIV)
>
> Beyond all question, the **mystery** of *godliness* is great: He appeared in a body, was vindicated by the Spirit, was seen by angels, was preached among the nations, was believed on in the world, was taken up <u>*in glory*</u>. (1 Timothy 3:16 NIV)
>
> Listen, I tell you a **mystery**: We will not all sleep, but <u>*we will all be changed*</u>— (1 Corinthians 15:51 NIV)
>
> But we all, with open face beholding as in a glass *the glory of the Lord*, <u>*are* changed *into the same image* from *glory to glory*</u>, even as by the Spirit of the Lord. (2 Corinthians 3:18 KJV)

Isaiah 43:7 says man was created for God's glory. Traditionally, the church has taken that to mean that man was created so that God would be praised for His excellent creation or to bring God glory. However, if you read it again in context, the word "*for*" carries not only the meaning of "to bring glory to", but *also* the meaning of *"created on purpose in order **to live in**"* his glory. Selah.

Look again at 2 Corinthians 3:18. It is His will that we all *are changed into the same image, the image of the glory of the Lord.* His Glory is the place where we were originally *designed to live*, spirit, soul, and physical body, connected to and in *fellowship* with God. But Christians, as a whole body, have not yet moved very far *from the glory* of salvation. According to the Word, He desired that we be changed, reconciled, *to the glory* of living, existing, and receiving our every provision, *In Him,* like He originally intended.

God is Life. He is The Provider, The Healer, The Deliverer.

Beloved, His intent was and is and always will be for us to abide in *ever-increasing* glory! There is the answer: Christians suffer sickness, disease, and lack because they are not doing that! They are not living in, abiding in, dwelling in, His Glory. In Him, in His Glory is the source of power, light and life itself, health to our body and peace for our mind.

When Christ died, the sin debt was paid in full. But there was more. When Christ was resurrected, we were reconciled! We are no longer separated from God. We can commune with Him in His glory once again as it was in the beginning!

It is ours to partake of by grace through faith in Christ. We were *created to*, and now through Christ have been made *able to*, **live** *in* His glory…continually.

Consider this: Ephesians 5:27 (KJV) says He reconciled us in order "that he might present it to himself a glorious church, not having spot, or wrinkle, or any such thing; but that it should be holy and without blemish." This intimate fellowship, abiding, in the glory of God is the way we lay hold of the fullness and full measure of His provision. It is the way we are transfigured into His image. It is also the way we become the glorious church that is the testimony to the world of His love and of Christ. It must happen here on earth or the world would never see it. *Selah.*

THE PICTURE OF HEALTH®
DAILY POWER PLAN™
Day 99

1 Corinthians 11:26-28 (Amplified Bible)

> For every time you eat this bread and drink this cup, you are representing and signifying and proclaiming the fact of the Lord's death until He comes [again].
>
> So then whoever eats the bread or drinks the cup of the Lord in a way that is unworthy [of Him] will be guilty of [profaning and sinning against] the body and blood of the Lord.
>
> Let a man [thoroughly] examine himself, and [only when he has done] so should he eat of the bread and drink of the cup.

Selah (pause and reflect):

"Koinonia". Intimate fellowship. Communion. Communion, beloved, is the way we lay hold of the fullness and full measure of His provision. It is the way we are transfigured into His image. It is the way we become the glorious church that is the testimony to the world of His love and of Christ.

Right before Jesus gave himself on the cross for our sins, he gave his disciples these instructions found in Luke, chapter 22, but also in Paul's account in 1 Corinthians 11:23-25 (NIV):

> For I received from the Lord what I also passed on to you: The Lord Jesus, on the night he was betrayed, took bread, and when he had given thanks, he broke it and said, "This is my body, which is for you; do this in remembrance of me." In the same way, after supper he took the cup, saying, "This cup is the new covenant in my blood; do this, whenever you drink it, in remembrance of me."

Most people think "communion" is a religious service where Christians partake of bread and wine in remembrance of the body and blood of Jesus. Communion is a *holy* sacrament, but it is also *so much more than man has made of it*! It *is* remembering and reverencing Him for giving his body and blood for us, but it is also remembering *why* and *for what purpose* he did it.

In John 14:6, Jesus said, "I am the way and the truth and the life. No one comes to the Father except through me." When He held up the bread and the cup to his disciples, He was saying this to them all over again. He was teaching them to remember, attaching it to something they would do numerous times every day, every time they ate and drank, and most especially when they "communed" together in celebration of God's love.

He wasn't teaching them another religious ritual like that of the Pharisees.

He was showing us Himself.

Beloved, he was giving us the wisdom and the way to remember why He gave his life (because the Father so loved the world), and the reason for His shed blood and bruised and pierced body (as payment for our sin), and the result of His resurrection (our reconciliation to the Father).

He was telling them to remember that *His* death and resurrection established *our* communion, our intimate union, with the LORD GOD, Jehovah Elohim, The Way (Jesus Christ, The Son), The Truth (Holy Spirit), and The Life (God, The Father)!

So, now seeing it more clearly, how do we partake of it more intimately? How do we move from the glory of Salvation to the glory of complete provision where every spiritual, emotional, and physical need is met and our physical health is sustained continually by the power of God?

These are Jesus' words:

> Abide in me, and I in you. As the branch cannot bear fruit of itself, except it abide in the vine; no more can ye, except ye abide in me. I am the vine, ye are the branches: *He that abideth in me, and I in him, the same bringeth forth much fruit*: for without me ye can do nothing. *If a man abide not in me, he is cast forth as a branch, and is withered*; and men gather them, and cast them into the fire, and they are burned. *If ye abide in me, and my words abide in you,* **ye shall ask what ye will, and it shall be done unto you**. (John 15:4-6 KJV)

You see, anyone who comes to God through Christ can ask and receive provision from God! So why don't more Christians have what they need to be healthy and whole and prosperous in every way? The problem is *not* that *He* doesn't *provide*! It is that *we don't abide*! We won't *stay in position* to receive it or retain it! He continually offers it and we repeatedly walk right out of His presence, leaving His provision behind.

Our "Power Verse™" today says to "let a man examine himself". This means to check yourselves, to observe, to study, to scrutinize, and to judge yourselves in the Light of the Word (not as compared to anyone else and not judging anyone else). If we sincerely look into His Word, we will find what is blocking the effectual work of the glory in our lives:

> I am come a light into the world, that whosoever believeth on me *should not abide in darkness.* (John 12:46 KJV)

> Be ye not unequally yoked together with unbelievers: for what fellowship hath righteousness with unrighteousness? and *what communion hath light with darkness?* (2 Corinthians 6:14 KJV)

> If we claim to have fellowship with him yet walk in the darkness, we lie and *do not live by the truth.* (1 John 1:6 NIV)

> Since you died with Christ to the basic principles of this world, *why, as though you still belonged to it, do you submit to its rules?* (Colossians 2:20 NIV)

He has given us the way to believe in, receive of, and be sustained by His glory:

> ...if we *walk in the light,* **as** *he is in the light*, we have fellowship one with another, and the blood of Jesus Christ his Son cleanseth us from all sin. (1John 1:7 KJV)

> Whoever claims to live in him *must walk as Jesus did.* (1 John 2:6 NIV)

> Whoever loves his brother *lives in the light*, and there is nothing in him to make him stumble. (1 John 2:10 NIV)
>
> *No one who lives in him keeps on sinning.* No one who continues to sin has either seen him or known him. (1 John 3:6 NIV)
>
> *Those who obey his commands live in him,* and he in them. And this is how we know that he lives in us: We know it by the Spirit he gave us. (1John 3:24 NIV)

I want to share with you a portion of a message preached by Smith Wigglesworth. He lived from 1859 to 1947 and was deeply filled with the Spirit and power of God. These are his words from a message entitled, "Faith is the Substance of Things Hoped For":

> "The Holy Ghost wants us to clearly understand that we are a million times bigger than we know. No Christian in this place has any conception of what he or she is. My heart is so big that I want to look into your faces and tell you that if you only knew what you had, your bodies would scarcely be able to contain it. Oh, that God shall so bring us into divine attractiveness by his almightiness that the whole of our bodies shall wake up to the resurrection force, to the divine, inward flow of eternal power coursing through the human frame." (Excerpt from "The Anointing of His Spirit", Smith Wigglesworth, compiled and edited by Wayne Warner, published by Vine Books, © 1994 Wayne E. Warner)

Beloved, communion with God through Christ, like Jesus had with the Father (constant, intimate, fellowship, with no darkness at all) is His design, His desire, and His will for your life and mine. It is by faith that we believe He has provided this communion *and* by faith that we believe it *supplies all things necessary* for life and godliness. And, it is by faith that we lay hold those things! Philemon 1:6 says that…

>The *intimate union*, the "koinonia",
>of your *faith*
>
>***becomes effectual***
>
>by the *acknowledging* (believing and receiving) of *every good thing*
>
>which is in you in Christ Jesus.

The Picture of Health®
Daily Power Plan™
Day 100

Colossians 2: 6 (The Message)

My counsel for you is simple and straightforward: Just go ahead with what you've been given. You received Christ Jesus, the Master; now live him.

Selah (pause and reflect)

That is my closing Word for you, my dear friends. We've been through many weeks together and have taken many "power walks" with Him through His Word. Now it is time for each of us to take the truths He has revealed to us in His precious Word to the world to which we are called.

As you go into all the world, remember…it is the Lord Christ you are serving in every act of worship, whether in the spirit, the soul (mind, will, emotions), or the body. He *has* equipped you to do what He has called you to do. Be strong in the Lord and *the power of His might*.

May His peace be with you all and may all grace abound to you through faith in our Lord Jesus Christ!

Amen

Printed in the United States
204162BV00004B/10-15/A